the ultimate

natural beauty book

the ultimate
natural
beauty
book

100 gorgeous beauty products
to make easily at home

JOSEPHINE FAIRLEY

with photographs by
ANNIE HANSON

Kyle Cathie Limited

First published in Great Britain in 2004 by
Kyle Cathie Limited,
122 Arlington Road,
London NW1 7HP
general.enquiries@kyle-cathie.com
www.kylecathie.com

2 4 6 8 10 9 7 5 3 1

ISBN 1 85626 513 7

Stylist   Josephine Fairley
Editor   Stephanie Horner
Designer   Fran Rawlinson
Proof reader   Katie Joll
Indexer   Ursula Caffrey
Production   Sha Huxtable and Alice Holloway

A Cataloguing in Publication record for this title is available from
the British Library.

Colour reproduction by Sang Choy
Printed and bound in China by C&C Offset Printing Co Ltd

To the next generation of gorgeous girls – Fifi, Carson, Peaches, Pixie, Elvi, Roxy, Saba, Tiger, Little Roxy and Peggy – and to two handsome young men: Paris and Mars. But most especially this book is dedicated to Lily (Evans), for her invaluable and unfailingly cheerful help at all times as lighting assistant, gofer, backdrop-painter, tester – and model.

contents

introduction

Despite everything the billion-dollar cosmetics giants like to tell us, making skincare and haircare couldn't be easier. Now, I'm no Nigella Lawson or Jamie Oliver. (Let alone a three-star Michelin chef.) But there's a simple truth: if you can make a salad dressing or brew a cup of tea – or melt chocolate in a double-boiler into a pool of yumminess – then the world of truly, totally, 100 percent natural cosmetics is wide open to you.

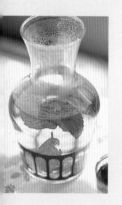

Natural beauty care is something I've been passionately interested in for as long as I can remember. My first attempt to make cosmetics involved rose petals and water, aged around three, and was actually intended as a **magical** concoction for the fairies I was convinced were living under our weeping silver birch. But today there's a different reason why, whenever I can, I make my own cosmetics: **I prefer to know exactly what I'm putting on my skin** – just as I choose very carefully what I put in my mouth. (Which is why I grow, buy and eat exclusively organic food.) Increasingly, that's the message I'm getting from other women, too: we want a 'cleaner' lifestyle. And the penny is dropping that **even so-called natural cosmetics aren't always as natural** as they're cracked up to be. They may still contain a high percentage of chemicals – and many of us are making a lifestyle change to reduce our overall 'chemical load', because we're unsure about the future impact that the untested daily 'cocktail' of food additives, preservatives, prescription and over-the-counter drugs, pesticides and synthetic fragrances might have on our health, somewhere down the line.

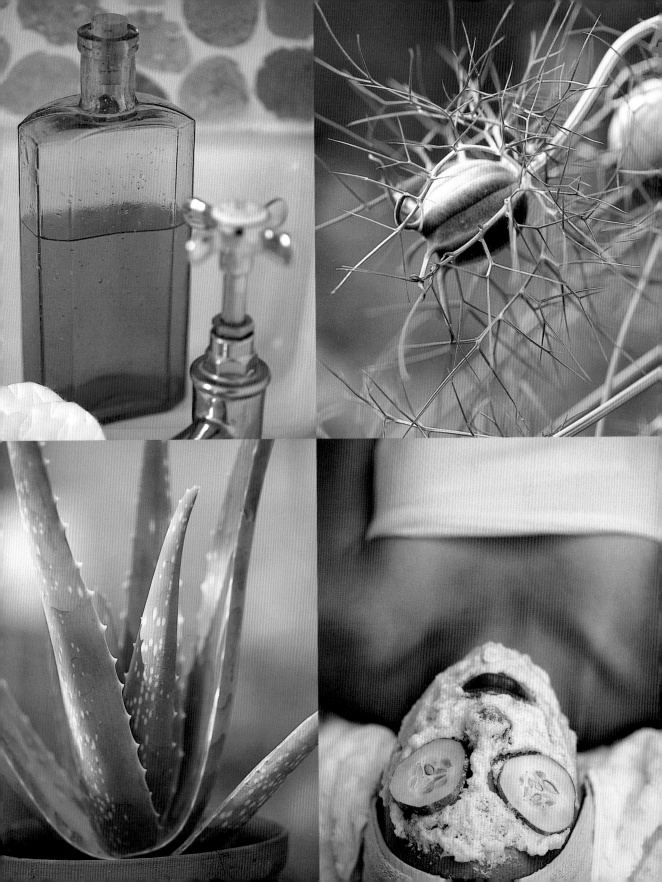

By harnessing the power of plants and herbs yourself to make your own cosmetics using natural ingredients, you'll also know you're getting the **full impact of plant goodness** – benefits which have been understood by 'wise women' down the centuries and chronicled by famous herbalists, among them Culpeper and Gérard. **The truly botanical beauty world is full of skin-saving ingredients**: rose, for anti-ageing; sage, as a deodorant; antioxidant-rich marigold, to soothe troubled complexions. (**Perfect in a world where so many women complain of sensitive skins**.)

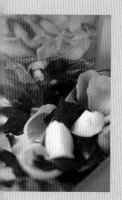

In fact, my own interest in making cosmetics at home has also been driven by increasing sensitivity to synthetic cosmetics – what I call 'beauty editor's skin', a response to having to regularly assault my skin with cream-after-new-cream, as part of my research. And, while so-called 'natural' cosmetics you buy in a beauty hall might well list some active botanicals on the label, the reality is that most are highly processed and their 'natural' powers completely diluted by the time they hit the shelves.

You don't have to be a lady of leisure to make your own cosmetics, either: it's possible to whip up a cleanser, toner and moisturiser (plus a mask, to boot) far, far more quickly than it is to cook a three-course dinner. Since I began seriously experimenting with making my own cosmetics as a teenager, it's never ceased to amaze me how **effective** these home-made versions are, how little time it takes to make them, and how much **fun** I can have, creating and inventing.

I'm not pretending there's no place for shop-bought cosmetics – especially when there's too much to do in too little time, and now that there are certified-organic cosmetics on the market. (The Soil Association, in the UK, and Ecocert, in France, both certify cosmetics that meet their strict criteria, and you'll see their symbols on cosmetics available worldwide.) But there are some amazing alternatives to much of what you'll find at the beauty counter that are **simple to make** – and heaven to use. And for this book, I have stuck to the very easiest recipes, which even someone who can barely boil an egg can create…

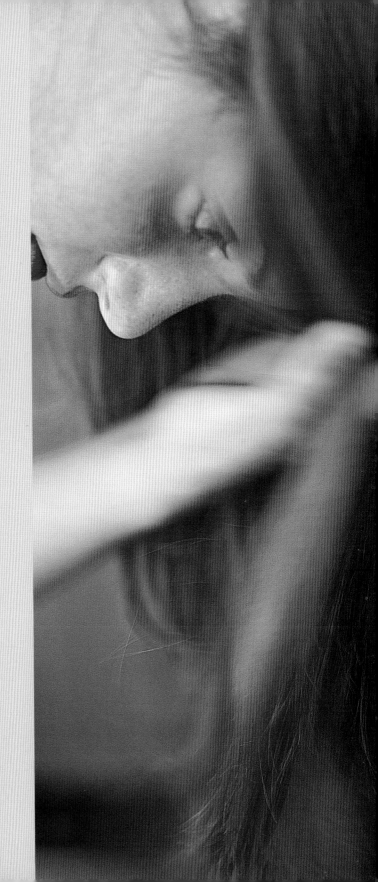

One of the big revelations, when you make your own cosmetics, is how much **money you can save**. (Especially if you're using store-cupboard staples such as olive oil or eggs in your recipes.) I reckon that a whole year's supply of home-made bath, body and hair treats will probably **cost you less than a single fancy jar of branded anti-ageing cream**.

But don't expect the cosmetics you make always to look, feel – or indeed last as long – as those you can buy in a marbled beauty hall. The lotions, creams and other skin and hair treats in this book are designed to be made and used straight away or in other cases, to have a shelf-life of a few weeks or possibly months, then be made afresh, to optimise the effectiveness of the plant ingredients. Some recipes feature such natural preservatives as wheatgerm oil or grapefruit seed extract – but what you definitely won't find in any recipe is the long list of synthetic preservatives you'll encounter on the label of most store-bought cosmetics. (Those preservatives will keep commercial cosmetics on the shelf in a state of 'suspended animation'

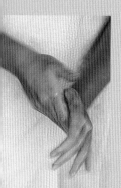

for up to three years, and they are there as much to protect the manufacturer from complaints that the product has an odd colour or texture, as to 'protect' the beauty-hound.) By making cosmetics from fresh, you can also help to **optimise the effectiveness of the plant ingredients**.

Meanwhile, why am I calling this the 'ultimate' natural beauty book? Because virtually all the recipes and formulations in this book contain **ingredients which can actually be grown at home** – if you've the time, the space (even a window box or a back yard) and the inclination. And if that part sounds way too difficult, time-consuming or knit-your-own-muesli, for your lifestyle, there's a short-cut: the herbal, fruit, vegetable and plant ingredients can all be bought from a natural foodstore, by mail order – or even in the supermarket. (For some of the recipes, though, you will need other simple ingredients which you can readily source from a health shop: beeswax, base oils – and perhaps some essential oils, too, if you want to make your lotions and potions

smell ravishing – see RESOURCES, pp.154–7.) Personally, I'd recommend using **organic whenever it's available**. To me, that's part of the point: to ensure what I put on my skin is as pure as possible. Which is why I grow almost all the plant ingredients I've used in this book in my own organic back garden.

I certainly think life is too short to stuff a mushroom. (Sometimes, it's too short to dust the hall table, frankly.) But with everything I've learned about beauty over the past fifteen years, I don't think it's too short to **discover the pleasure of making your own cosmetics**. Wise women (and men) of the twenty-first century, there's a garden of gorgeousness out there. **Have fun** exploring it…

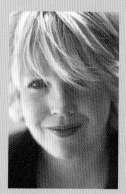

Josephine Fairley

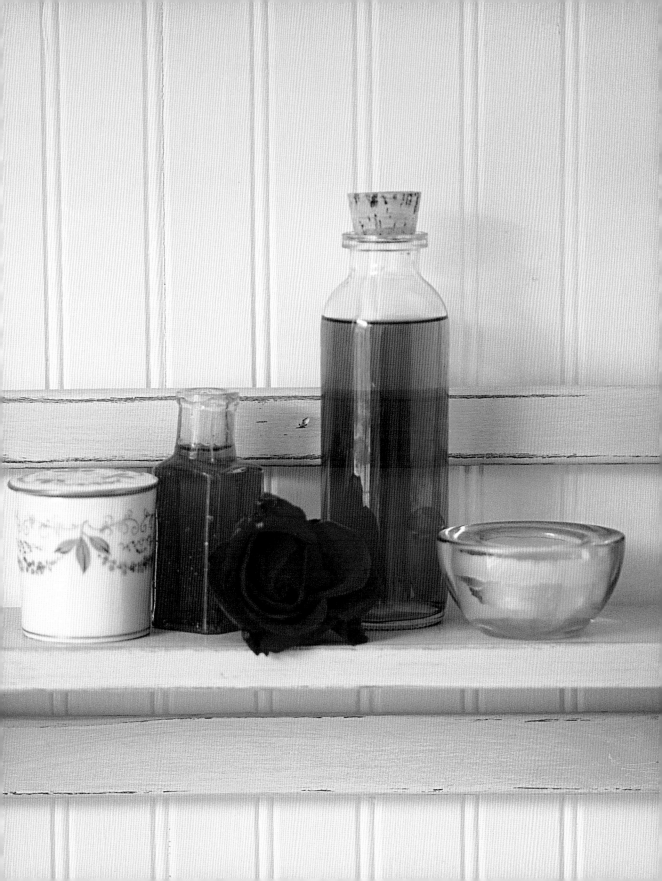

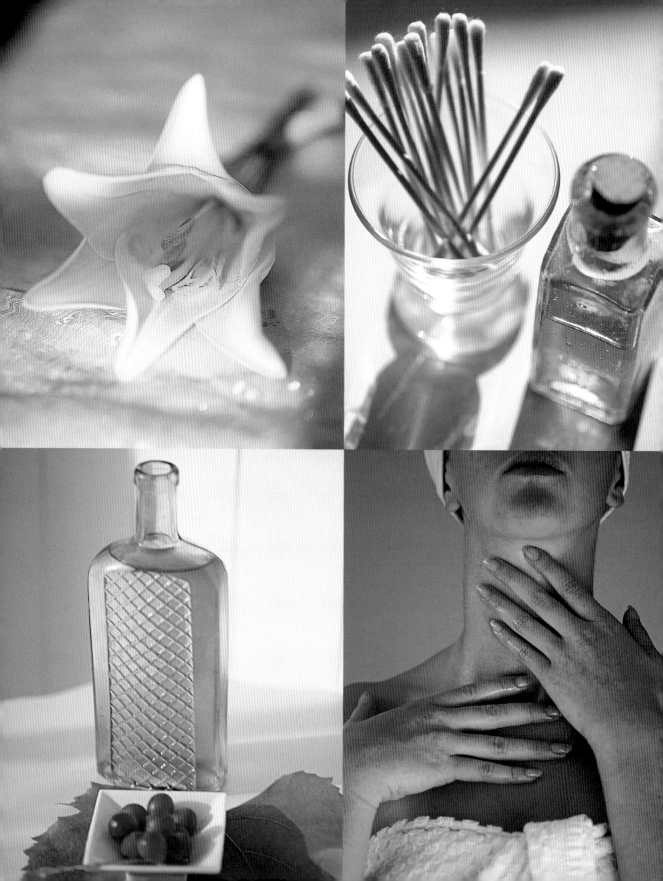

face

Most cosmetics are packed with synthetic ingredients – some of which have a **health question mark** over them, while others are linked with the **increase in reported sensitivity**. (Sixty-three percent of us claim to have sensitive skin, according to insiders.) But when it comes to daily skincare, **nature has all the answers** – helping to control oiliness or dryness, or to defy time. Nature can soothe frazzled complexions beautifully, too – as well as stop break-outs in their tracks. **So step inside the skincare garden**…

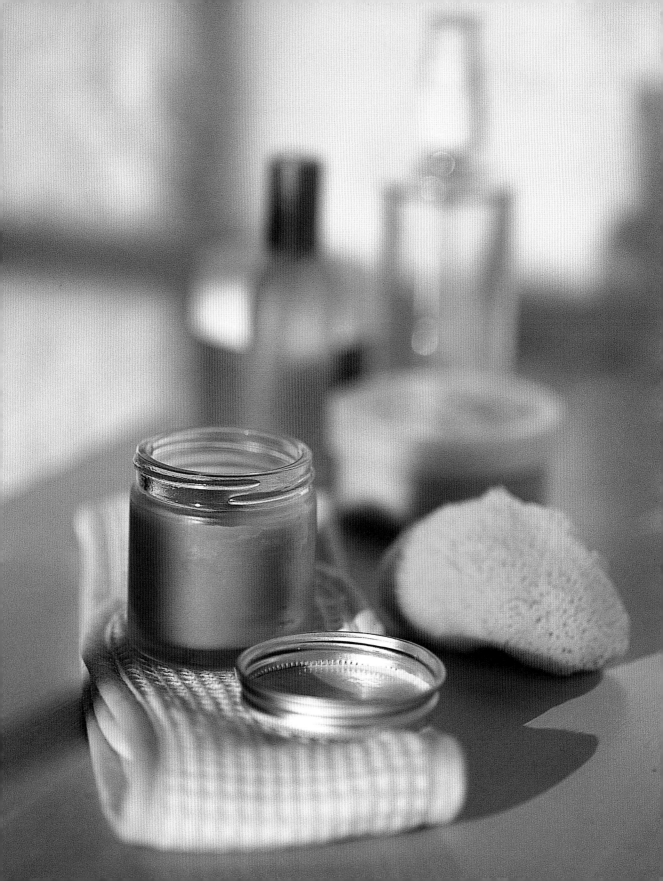

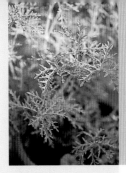

GERANIUM
Pelargonium odoratissimum

How cosmetics smell influences their pleasure factor. So scented-leaf geraniums are invaluable in concocting beauty treats: their rose-like fragrance makes bath powders, balms and creams bliss for the senses. These are tender perennial plants, which need to be overwintered on a windowsill or in a greenhouse. In commercial cosmetics production, geranium is distilled to obtain geraniol, a volatile oil given off when you rub the leaves.

Which geranium do you choose? There are so many varieties, so go for the one whose scent most appeals to you. My favourite is 'Attar of Roses', though I also love *Pelargonium graveolens*, which is also rose-scented; to me, that will always be the smell of my grandmother, who grew them in a sheltered porch outside her back door. The leaves will infuse a base oil – anything from olive oil, sunflower, grapeseed, to avocado – or a body powder (see recipe, p. 107) with their *faux*-rosiness. I also believe rose geranium essential oil should be in every at-home-beauty-creator's portfolio of essential oils, for deliciously scenting all kinds of lotions and potions.

geranium cleansing balm

To use this miraculous, make-up-melting cleanser, massage it thoroughly into your face and remove with a muslin washcloth or flannel that's been dunked in hot water; repeat until your face is completely clean.

75ml (3fl oz) extra virgin olive oil
10g (¹/₂oz) beeswax granules or grated beeswax
12 fresh scented geranium leaves
10 drops geranium essential oil

Heat the olive oil and the beeswax in the top of a double-boiler until melted (see p. 153). Place the leaves in the bottom of a sterilised, heatproof glass jar (which has a lid or cork) and as soon as the oil and beeswax have melted, pour them over the leaves. Seal and leave for 3 weeks to infuse the mixture with geranium-ness; then scoop everything out and reheat in a double-boiler. Strain through kitchen paper or muslin to remove the leaves and when the mixture has cooled very slightly, add 10 drops of geranium essential oil, and stir, before transferring to a sterilised wide-necked jar.

Dry skins also love... Emollient and hydrating plants and herbs (chamomile, comfrey, fennel, elderflower, marshmallow, orange blossom, rose and violet...)

TIP

Dry skin can sometimes be the result of a vitamin B deficiency. Great sources include goat's milk, wholegrain rice, sunflower seeds, sprouted seeds, oats, yeast, bran and yeast extract.

home-made rosewater

Personally, I don't believe in toners – I think they're too harsh for skin. Dry skins in particular can be stripped of vital oils by harsh toners. But most of us like the feeling of sweeping away the last traces of a cleanser with a fresh lotion. This 'home-made' rosewater is a cheat – but frankly, it's all the toner or freshener a dry skin needs. To make genuine rosewater you need distilling equipment – and several hours; the plant's oils are evaporated into steam, cooled – and the result is pure rosewater. But you can easily create a great 'fake' rosewater on the stove.

Freshly picked, unsprayed rose petals

Pack the top of a double-boiler (see p. 153) half-full with the rose petals. Cover with filtered, mineral or rainwater. Put a lid on the pan and simmer over a very, very gentle heat for 1 hour. Remove the bowl and allow to cool before squishing the petals between your hands to squeeze out all the liquid. Discard the used petals and repeat, using fresh petals in the original water. Cool, then strain the water into a sterilised bottle or jar. You only get a small quantity, though by now it should be smelling sweetly of roses. This should last for 1–2 weeks – longer in the fridge – so you only need to make a small quantity at a time.

rich rose moisturiser

The perfect, rich-textured, sumptuously scented night-time moisturiser for thirsty skin. If you like, add 10 drops of frankincense essential oil as well as the rose. Frankincense is renowned for its anti-ageing powers.

2 large handfuls of fresh, scented rose petals
50ml (2fl oz) sweet almond oil or extra virgin olive oil
5g (¼oz) beeswax granules or grated beeswax
1 teaspoon wheatgerm oil
15 drops rose essential oil

Pack the rose petals in a wide-necked glass jar and cover with sweet almond oil. Bruise the petals with a spoon in the jar, to start the maceration process, and seal the jar. Position it where it can absorb sunlight daily (a south-facing windowsill is just perfect), to speed up the infusion process. After 3 weeks, strain off the rose-infused oil.

Heat the beeswax in the sweet almond oil in the top of a double-boiler (see p. 153) until melted. Remove from heat and allow to cool slightly before adding the wheatgerm oil and rose essential oil. Cool for a further 1–2 minutes then pour into a sterilised glass jar to set thoroughly. The mixture will harden, but it emulsifies when you touch it.

TIP

Wheatgerm acts as a natural preservative; you don't need to keep this refrigerated. If you can't find wheatgerm oil, you can pierce wheatgerm capsules, available from natural foodstores, and measure into a teaspoon.

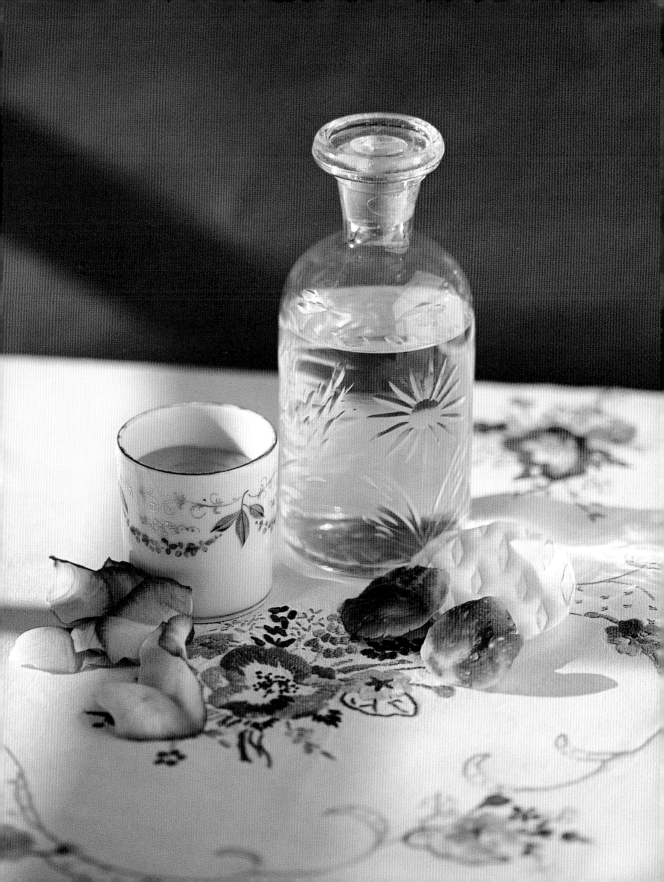

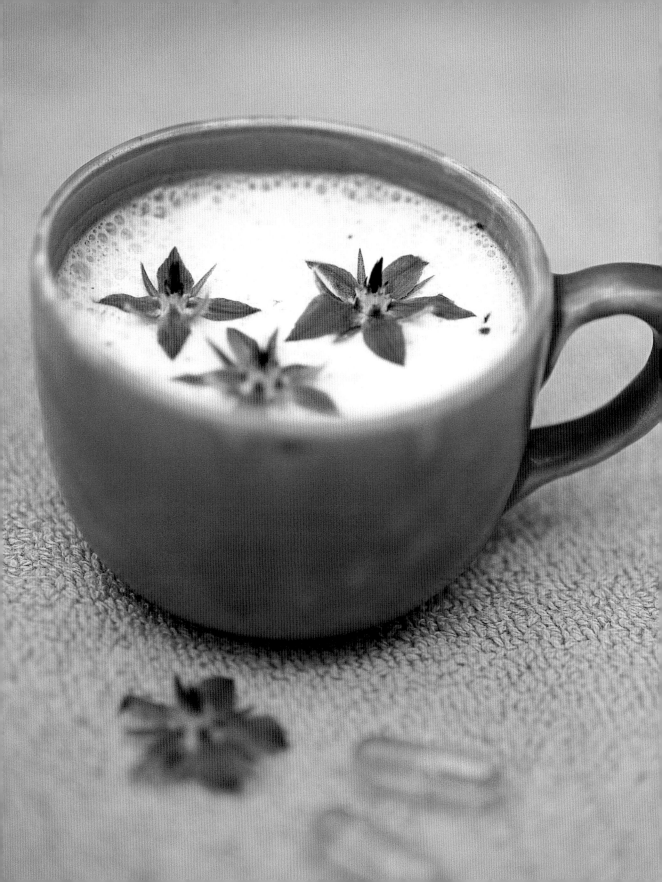

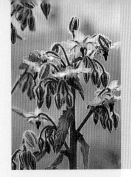

BORAGE
Borago officinalis

This pretty, blue-flowered, sun-loving plant is a real hussy: once you have it in your garden, it puts itself about all over the place (creating lovely, unexpected plant combinations, in my experience). Borage also has the advantage of a three-month flowering season, in high summer. The name of the plant comes from the Latin *burra*, or hairy garment, because the leaves and stems are almost bristly. But appearances can be deceptive: the juice of the plant is soothing to damaged or irritated tissues. The leaves can be made into an infusion, or tea (see p. 153) and used to bathe the eyes. The flowers are also gorgeously chic in salads – but may be much more than decorative: eaten like that, according to legendary herbalist Gérard, 'they do exhilarate and make the mind glad.'

TIP

The best way to remove all masks is with a clean muslin washcloth or even a good old face flannel; these swoosh away the last traces of the mask along with any dead skin cells that are ready to come away, leaving skin beautifully bright.

starflower mask

Full credit to my husband Craig Sams for discovering this particular miracle-worker. It is my all-time favourite mask – I love how the borage flowers, which I add in season, speckle it with gorgeous flecks of lapis lazuli blue, and how it softens and 'plumps' my dry skin.

2 capsules starflower (borage flower) oil
50g (2oz) aloe vera flesh
30ml (1fl oz) plain yogurt
10 fresh borage flowers (in season)

Snip the starflower oil capsules, and squeeze out the oil. Then blend everything together (aloe vera flesh is quite hard to blend, so I use an electric herb chopper to zoosh all the ingredients). Massage the mixture into the skin of your face and neck, avoiding the eyes and mouth area, whereupon the most extraordinary thing happens: within 15 minutes, your complexion will have soaked up almost all of the mask, and look plumped-up and younger. Rinse well with warm water, pat dry and moisturise as usual.

apricot softening mask

This mask couldn't be simpler – or more nourishing.

2 fresh apricots
1 teaspoon avocado oil

Blanch the apricots in just-boiled water for 1 minute to make it easy to peel off the skins. Slice to remove the stones, then mash the flesh to a smooth pulp, adding the oil in a trickle. Spread onto the face, avoiding the eyes and mouth area, and relax for 20 minutes while the softening ingredients get to work. Rinse well with warm water, pat dry and moisturise as usual.

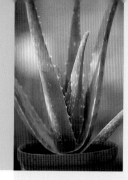

aloe vera cleanser

According to beauty lore, this is pretty close to what Cleopatra – Egypt's own beauty queen – used to cleanse her face. (Including that famous eyeliner!) Either peel your own aloe leaves, or buy aloe vera gel from a natural foodstore.

30ml (1fl oz) aloe vera gel
50ml (2fl oz) olive oil
30ml (1fl oz) rosewater
4 drops rose essential oil
2 drops grapefruit seed extract

Blend all the ingredients together in a food processor and decant into a small bottle. Ideally, keep in the fridge. Shake before use, as the ingredients may separate. Massage into your face and neck and remove with either a muslin wash cloth (my preference) or plain water.

dandelion skin tonic

This acts as a general daily pick-you-up for normal skins and can be used to sweep away the last traces of cleanser.

Generous handful of dandelion leaves
2 heaped tablespoons fresh thyme leaves (and flowers, if you like)
  or 1 tablespoon dried leaves
300ml (¹/₂ pint) boiling filtered, mineral or rainwater
1 tablespoon witch hazel
2 drops grapefruit seed extract

Infuse the dandelion flowers and thyme in the boiling water just as if you were making a tea (see p. 153); leave to cool for 20 minutes. Strain through a sieve and add the witch hazel. Lastly, add the drops of grapefruit seed extract and shake well.

ALOE VERA
Aloe barbadensis

Everyone needs an aloe near the kitchen window. This ancient plant, originating in Africa, is mentioned in the Bible – even depicted on Egyptian tombs. The tough-looking spikes slice surprisingly easily to reveal a soft, shiny, cooling, gel-like sap – ultra-soothing for burns, scalds and sunburn. Fifty years ago, it was discovered that patients with facial X-ray burns treated with fresh aloe vera juice healed surprisingly fast, without scarring. (For serious burns, of course, you should always head for A & E.) Recent studies indicate that aloe vera is able to enhance or accelerate cell growth in the skin.

To harness aloe's healing power, cut off 5 cm (2 inches) of leaf, slice in half and apply the cut side to the affected area; as the gel dries it 'seals' the skin with a protective, healing covering. Or, simply peel the aloe and almost moosh it into the skin. (Avoid the greenish/brown juice of the rind, though, as this part can actually irritate.) In home-made creams and lotions, aloe vera creates a gel-like consistency which calms troubled skins.

Aloe seems to thrive on neglect, in my experience – over-watering is fatal. It's tender too: bring it indoors in cold months. But if you don't have your own plant, gel or juice is available from health food stores, although it's less 'gel-like' than that from a plant you grow yourself. Harvest the leaves from the outside of the plant as these are its mature leaves, and yield the most gel. It will regenerate from the inside out.

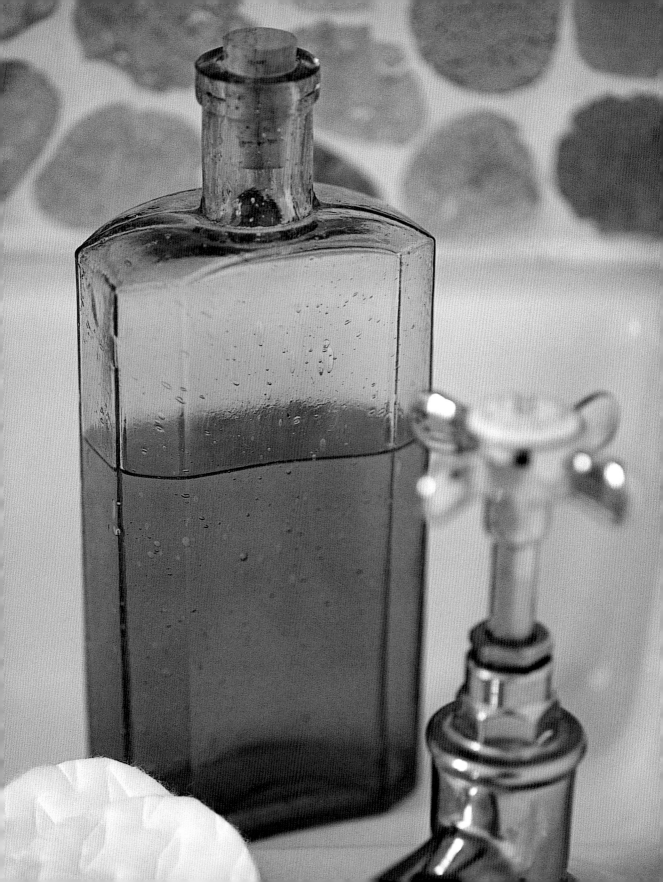

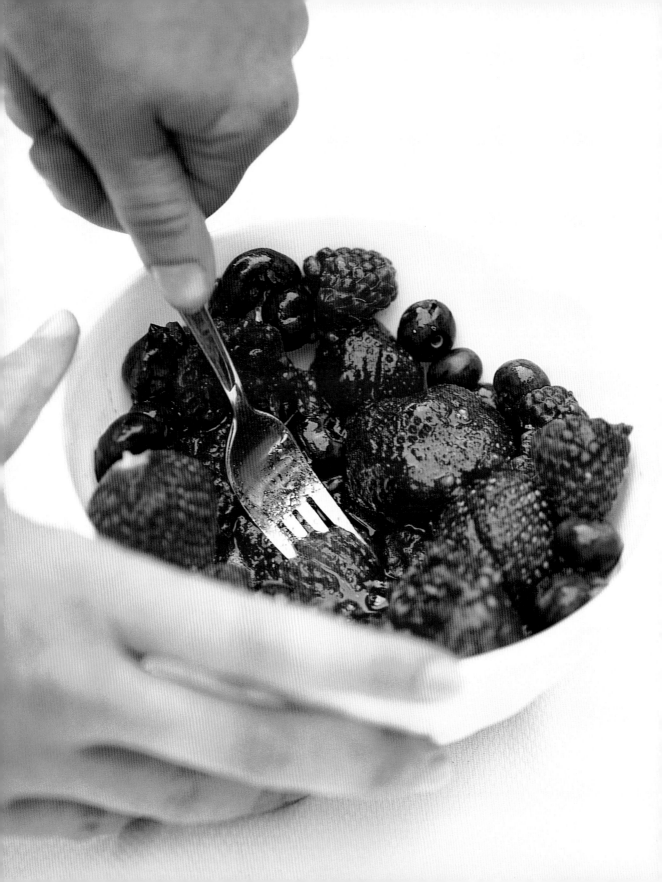

fruit-bowl facial

Fruit acids – from fresh fruits – are instantly skin-brightening. Simply use whichever luscious, fresh soft fruits you have to hand.

25g (1oz) finely ground oatmeal
25g (1oz) finely ground almonds
50g (2oz) soft fruits or vegetables of your choice
    (strawberries, raspberries, apricots, peach, plums,
    blueberries, cucumber, lettuce or tomatoes),
    chopped and mashed
Filtered, mineral or rainwater

Mix the dry ingredients in a bowl and stir well. Add the chopped and mashed fruit and/or vegetables and combine until the mixture is well blended. Stir in just enough water to form a soft paste. (Don't make it too runny.) Spread the mixture onto your face and massage in, avoiding the eyes and mouth area. Relax for 10–15 minutes, rinse well with warm water, pat dry and moisturise as usual.

Normal skins also love...

Almost anything! So if you're blessed with normal skin, thank your lucky stars. But you may find that in summer, your skin veers towards oiliness – and that in winter, it's dried by central heating and harsh weather. So look at the sections in this book for dry and for oilier skins, too; try the recipes and see how your skin responds.

lettuce face pack

Lettuce has an amazingly skin-softening effect and this is a fun – well, OK, hilarious – mask to try. You won't want to answer the door while wearing it! Just ponder this while you relax: according to Culpeper, the juice of lettuce, 'mixed or boiled with oil of roses, applied to the forehead and temples, procures sleep…'

8 lettuce leaves (any type – Little
    Gem are perfect), washed
300ml (1/2 pint) milk

Cook the washed lettuce leaves in the milk for 3 minutes – don't stir, as you want them to remain whole. Strain off the liquid and keep it aside. Layer the leaves over your pre-cleansed face, and relax for 20 minutes with them in place. Remove the leaves, and give skin a final swoosh with cotton wool pads soaked in the milk you put aside. Pat dry and moisturise as usual.

TIP

Strawberries are also great for sallow and oily skins; a *tisane* or infusion (see p. 153) of strawberry leaves can be applied as a freshener to calm overactive sebaceous glands.

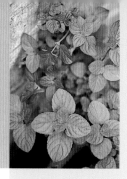

milk, cucumber and mint cleanser

This is wonderfully cooling and soothing on the skin. The milk is lightly hydrating, meanwhile, delivering a light veil of moisture that even oily skins need.

10 cm (2 inch) piece of cucumber
5 mint leaves
50ml (2fl oz) milk
2 drops grapefruit seed extract (or 4 drops of tincture of benzoin)

Peel the cucumber and chop it roughly. Remove the stalks and chop the mint leaves roughly. Place the cucumber and mint in a blender or food processor with the milk, and whizz until smooth. Pour the mixture into a pan and heat until simmering over a medium heat. Simmer for a further 2 minutes, and allow to cool. Strain through muslin (or a piece of kitchen paper). Pour the liquid into a sterilised bottle and add the grapefruit seed extract. Keep the cleanser in the fridge and use within a week.

MINT
Mentha piperata

Peppermint is a stimulating plant, which boasts mild antibacterial and antiseptic properties, making it perfect for 'problem' or oily skins, which have a tendency to break out. Peppermint helps to control the spread of bacteria on the skin's surface. It's also refreshing and invigorating – making skin tingle (in the best possible way). Fresh peppermint, dried peppermint and a few drops of peppermint essential oil are all useful for making cosmetics. As a quick-fix for tired feet, try a couple of drops of peppermint in a washing-up bowl of cool water and soak your feet for 10 minutes to put the spring back in your step.

Growing mint couldn't be easier. It's a positive hooligan, making a takeover bid for the surrounding area if you plant it in a flower bed. Instead, grow it in a pot – or a galvanised container, or bucket. Mint is thirsty, too. Water it often, and pick regularly. Personally (as someone who's constantly trying to kick caffeine), I like to grab a couple of sprigs, pour boiling water over them and steep, for a very refreshing, mind-clearing alternative to tea and coffee. (I don't drink it after 6 pm, though, as I find it has a tendency to keep me rather too awake.)

Some essential oils are best avoided by pregnant women and peppermint oil is one of them. To be on the safe side, avoid completely during the first 3 months of pregnancy or when taking homeopathic remedies.

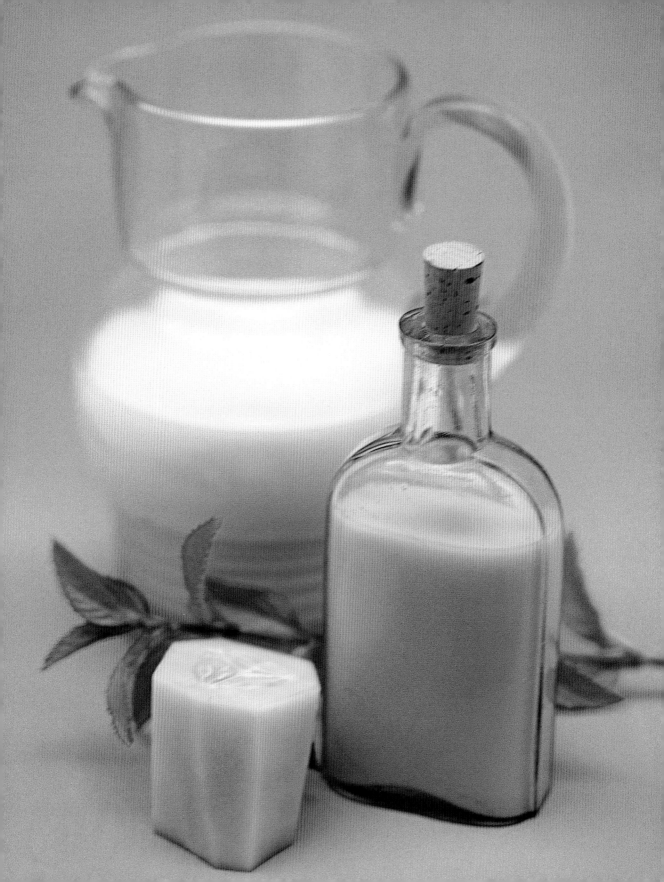

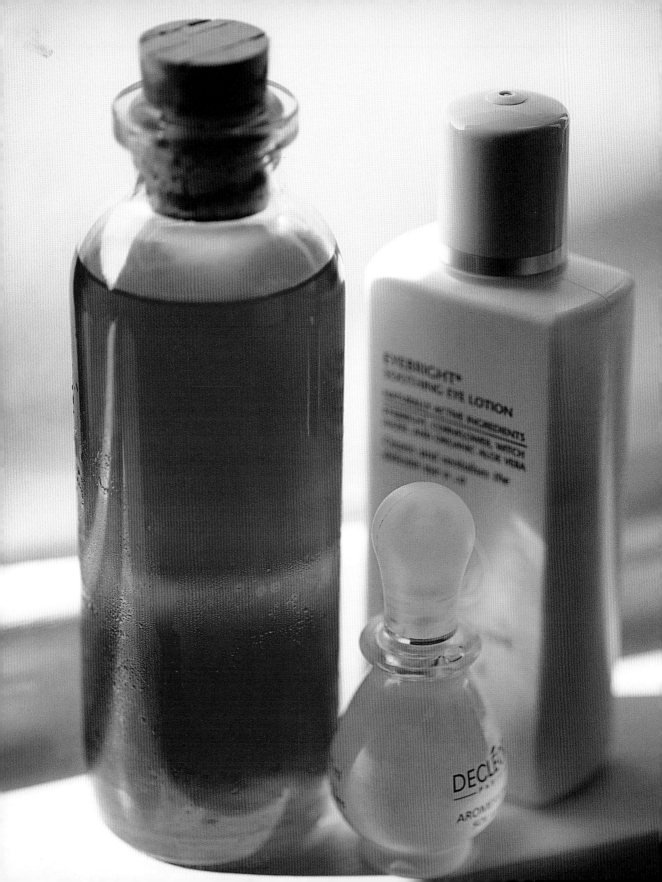

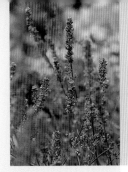

lavender skin tonic

LAVENDER
Lavandula officinalis, or
L. angustifolia

The name lavender may derive from the Latin *lavare*, meaning 'to wash', because ancient Romans valued the herb's scent and medicinal properties. It's definitely one of the most widely used fragrance elements in bath products today (even if that 'straight-from-Provence' scent is all too often synthesised rather than distilled from nature). Dried and infused into lotions, floral waters, and tonics lavender is antiseptic and toning, making it ideal for oily skins, or complexions prone to break-outs. Lavender essential oil, meanwhile, is almost the only essential oil which can be used neat on skin – I keep some in the kitchen and apply instantly to minor burns, with quite miraculous effect.

In the garden, lavender can be frost-tender, but it's usually quite happy in dry, sun-drenched conditions. It does, though, sulk if overwatered, and become woody and leggy unless trimmed immediately after flowering. (Cut the branches or stems to no more than 20cm (8 inches) or 15cm (6 inches) for younger plants.)

There are many different varieties of *Lavandula angustifolia*, with blooms that range from pale mauve to deepest blue. Choose whichever appeal to you most and grow anything from a potful to a long hedge, and harvest while in full flower – not just to create cosmetics but lavender sachets (great in the linen cupboard), and to bring back summer, heaped in china dishes around the house.

Lavender helps to 'normalise' sebum production, an excess of which manifests itself as spots. Ideally, keep this tonic in the fridge to preserve the pink colour which is part of its charm. If you don't, be aware that the colour will 'fade' in sunlight.

2 handfuls of lavender flowers (fresh or dried)
225ml (8fl oz) cider vinegar
700ml (1 1/4 pints) rosewater

Put the lavender flowers in the bottom of a screw-top jar, and add the liquid ingredients. Shake well, then put in the fridge. Allow the lavender to infuse the liquid for a week or two, and shake the jar once daily; the tonic will become a surprising rose colour. Strain the liquid and pour into a pretty bottle. Drench a cotton wool pad in the liquid and use to remove the last traces of cleanser. Make from fresh every few weeks.

Some people find their skin is sensitive to lavender, although for most of us, it lives up to its soothing reputation. As always, do the patch test first (see p. 145).

sage and yarrow
sinks-in-fast moisturiser

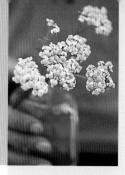

Tincture of benzoin and grapefruit seed extract act as natural preservatives, ensuring that this light, easily absorbed moisturiser keeps for a month or two without refrigeration.

1 tablespoon chopped fresh yarrow flowers or
*   2 teaspoons dried yarrow flowers*
1 tablespoon chopped fresh sage leaves or
*   2 teaspoons dried sage leaves*
125ml (4fl oz) filtered, mineral or rainwater
125ml (4fl oz) rosewater
2 tablespoons glycerine
1 tablespoon witch hazel
10 drops tincture of benzoin
2 drops grapefruit seed extract

Boil the herbs in the water (not the rosewater) in a pan to make a decoction (see p. 153); cover and simmer for 15 minutes. Allow to cool and then strain into a sterilised bottle. Add the rosewater, glycerine, witch hazel and the tincture of benzoin and grapefruit seed extract.

TIP

Be aware that commercial rosewater, bought in pharmacies, is often made with synthetic fragrance extracts, not distilled from roses. Buy from herbal and aromatherapy suppliers (I use Neal's Yard Remedies).

YARROW
Achillea millefolium

Yarrow is rich in compounds which suppress skin flare-ups, remove dead cells, slow down sebum production and help close pores – making it a wonder ingredient for greasy or problem skins, in particular. (A simple tea of yarrow works as a dandruff-blitzer, too.) With its fine, feathery, grey leaves and umbrellas of hundreds of gorgeous tiny, white or pink flowers, yarrow – also known as soldier's woundwort – looks really pretty in a sunny border, where it will flower uncomplainingly through even the driest summer. When I was writing this book, I also harvested yarrow which was growing wild on a bank near my house, so keep a look out for clumps. (One note of caution, though: prolonged use of this aromatic plant has, in a few cases, been linked with photosensitivity, so be conscious of that if you're planning to go in the sun, and always use an SPF15 zinc- or titanium-based sunblock, for protection – advice that applies to every skintype.)

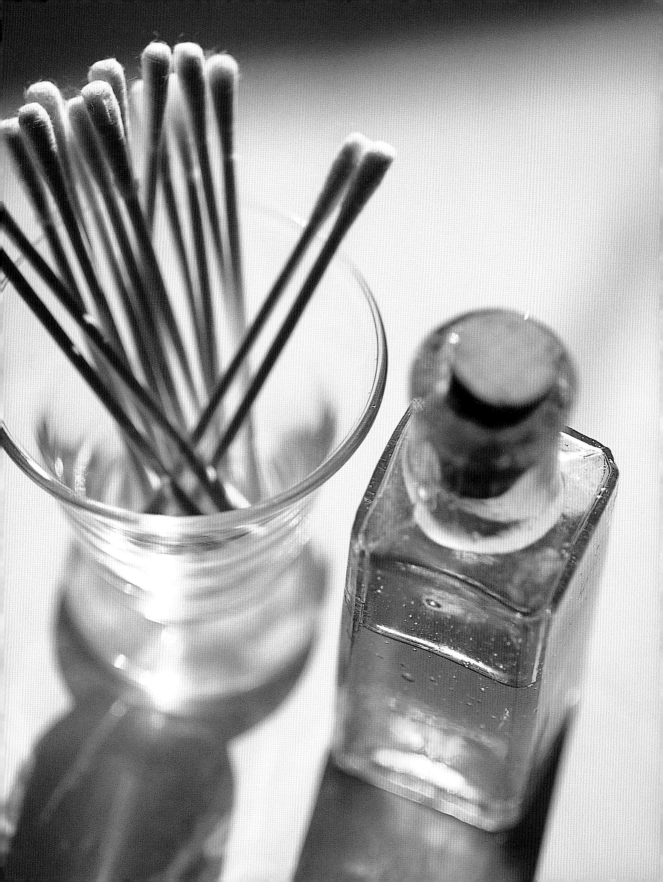

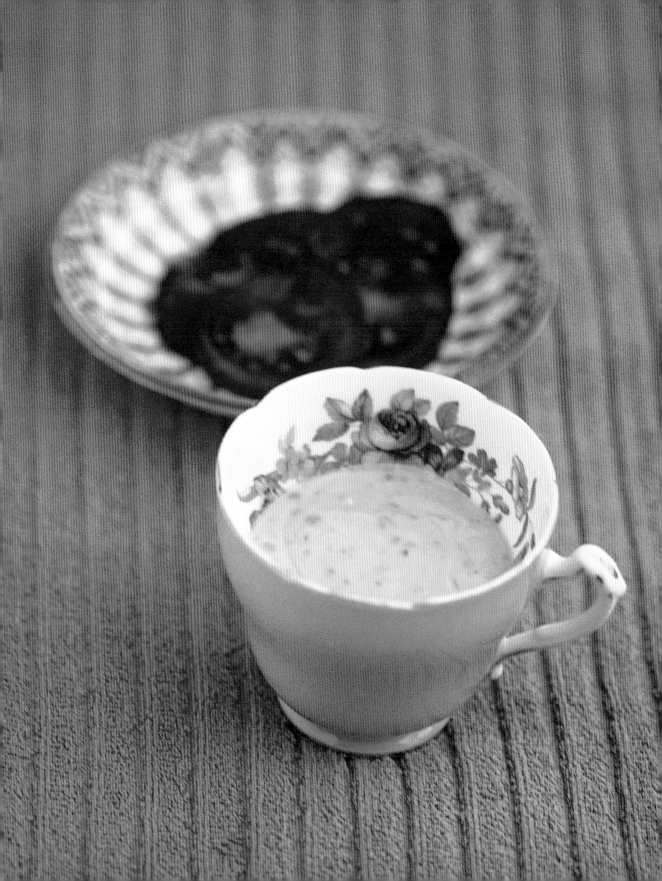

tomato face mask

The fruit acids in tomato are great for getting rid of blackheads and will brighten dull skin by gently loosening surface cells. This couldn't be simpler.

1 ripe tomato

Slice the tomato thickly but include some shaped or thin slices that will make it possible to cover your nose with tomato as well as your face. Lie down and apply the slices. Leave on for 10–15 minutes. Rinse well with warm water, pat dry but do not apply moisturiser to the nose zone (or other affected areas), as you'll only block the pores again.

mint and papaya facial

This (like the tomato mask) helps unclog blocked pores. The nicest thing about this treatment is that it starts with eating the papaya.

1 papaya
Handful of fresh peppermint leaves or
  2 tablespoons dried peppermint
2 drops peppermint essential oil

Halve the papaya, scoop out the seeds and flesh and reserve the peel. Put the peppermint in a large heat-proof bowl, pour over boiling water. Drape a towel over your head and steam your face above the bowl for a few minutes. Gently scrub skin with the inside of the papaya peel to slough away dead skin cells while conditioning skin with vitamins A and C.

raspberry skin brightener

The raspberries act as a gentle exfoliator, and the lactic acid in the yogurt has a brightening action.

2 tablespoons plain yogurt
75g (3oz) raspberries
3 drops sweet orange essential oil

Pulp the raspberries in a food processor then sieve the pulp over a bowl, reserving the flesh and seeds. (Drink the juice if you like – it's yummy!) Add the flesh and seeds to the yogurt and blend well; drop in the essential oil and stir again to mix. Apply to a cleansed face avoiding the eyes and mouth area. Leave on for 15 minutes and remove with a muslin washcloth dunked in warm water; rinse and pat dry.

Oily skins also love... Stimulating and antiseptic herbs like nettle, southernwood, thyme and rosemary; oatmeal, watercress …

TIP

Another mask option for spot-prone skins: whip 1 egg white, 1 teaspoon runny honey and 1–2 tablespoons oats to make a paste thick enough to spread on your face. This cleanses skin and also helps loosen blackheads. Leave on for 15 minutes and remove with a muslin washcloth dunked in warm water; rinse and pat dry.

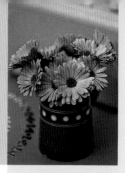

gentle marigold cleanser

Marigold (calendula) is one of the most healing and soothing treatments for delicate and sensitive skins. Use this as part of your nightly cleaning regime, to melt away make-up.

6 heads of marigold (calendula) flowers or
  20g (³/4oz) dried marigold flowers
10g (¹/2oz) cocoa butter
20g (³/4oz) beeswax granules
100ml (3¹/2fl oz) sweet almond oil or extra virgin olive oil

Remove all the petals from the marigold heads and place in a double-boiler (see p. 153). Add the other ingredients and gently heat until everything has melted, stirring gently. Continue to heat for about 5 minutes, then pour through a sieve into another bowl, stirring until the mixture is a little cooler but still runny. Transfer to a sterilised jar and seal when the mixture is fully cooled. Use within 6 months.

Even though the recipes in this section on sensitive skin are very gentle – and certainly don't cause any problems with my ultra-touchy skin – you should never introduce a whole new skincare regime in one go. Start with, say, the cleanser or moisturiser in this section, then give your skin a couple of weeks to adjust to it before introducing the next skin treat.

MARIGOLD
Calendula officinalis

Gorgeous orange flowers. Ridiculously easy to grow (they even colonise railway embankments and waste ground, in the wild, and seed themselves about without encouragement). One of nature's most healing, skin-soothing elements. Gentle enough for babies' skincare. What more could you ask?

Marigolds are rich in beta-carotene, antioxidants and salicylic acid. Hands, in particular, respond to marigolds' TLC – and when I get an eczema breakout (usually from using some just-launched wonder cream from a beauty company), I find that a calendula salve is the fastest way to settle my skin down again (though it's worth mentioning that very occasional adverse reactions have been reported – so remember your patch test, see p. 145, as always). Don't confuse this plant with the many bedding varieties of 'marigold' which are only useful in the flower border: look for the name calendula if you're buying seeds or young plants. Blondes can use marigold to add a gold tinge to their hair – just as they did in sixteenth-century Europe, when William Turner, Dean of Wells, wrote in *The New Herbal*: 'some women use to make their heyre yellow with the flowers of this herb, not being content with the natural colour which God hath given them.'

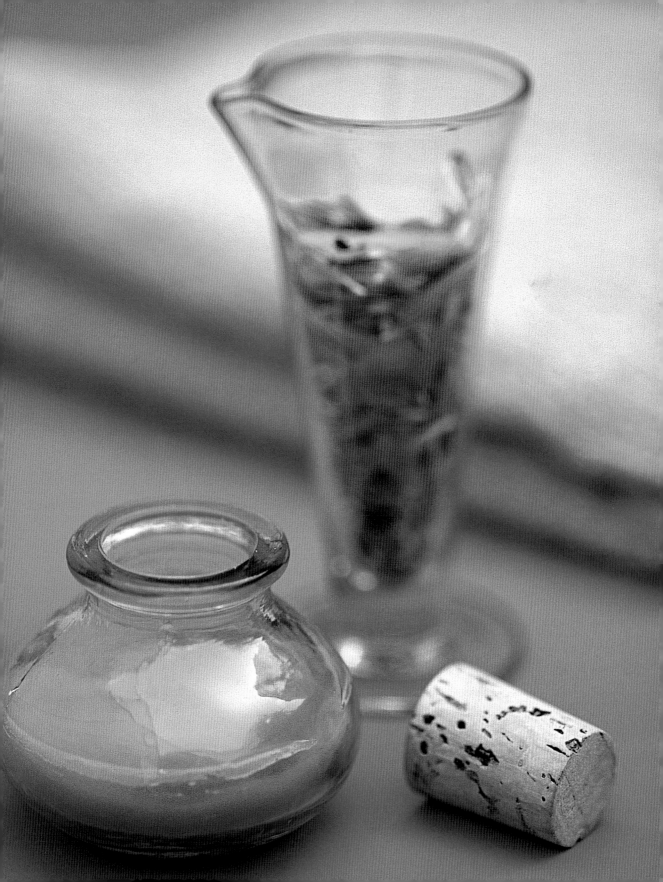

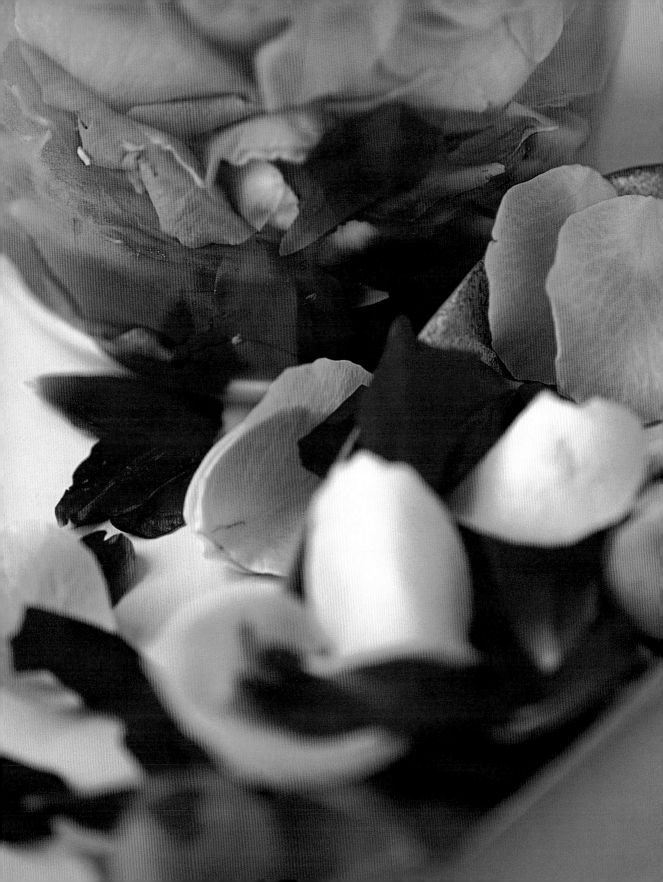

triple rose facial freshener

This facial freshener harnesses the gentle, skin-soothing power of roses – in triplicate. It makes a perfect morning cleanser, too.

25g (1 oz) dried rose petals
350ml (12fl oz) rosewater
50 ml (2fl oz) cider vinegar
2 drops rose essential oil

Put the rose petals in a bottle or jar and pour the vinegar and rosewater over. Add the drops of rose essential oil. Seal and leave to steep for 3 weeks in a cool dark place. Strain the liquid and pour into a sterilised bottle. You can either spritz this onto your face as a freshener, or apply with a cotton ball after you've cleansed.

TIP

If you suffer from sensitive skin, try treating it from the inside out with this skin-calming tea:

4 parts dandelion root and leaves (dried), 2 parts dried nettle, 1 part dried rosehip. Put 1 teaspoon of the mixed herbs in 225ml (8fl oz) boiling water, and drink 2 cups before meals, twice a day, for 6 weeks.

chamomile comfort cream

The first time I made this, my stepdaughter Rima declared that this was the best skin cream she'd ever used – it's gentle, nourishing and altogether luscious.

1 tablespoon dried chamomile flowers
150ml (1/4 pint) water
100ml (3 1/2fl oz) extra virgin olive oil
1 tablespoon runny honey
10g (1/2oz) beeswax
2 tablespoons vegetable glycerine
2 drops chamomile essential oil
2 drops calendula essential oil

Put the chamomile and water in a pan and bring to the boil; cover and simmer for 5 minutes to make a herbal decoction (see p. 153). Leave to cool, then strain off and discard the herbs. Place the oil, honey and beeswax in the top of a double-boiler and slowly add the glycerine; melt gently on a low heat and keep stirring. Remove from the heat and beat in the herbal decoction with a hand whisk or blender. Add the essential oils and stir again. Transfer to a sterilised jar or pot and cover when completely cold. Use within 2 months.

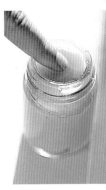

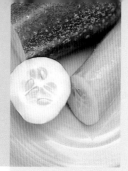

cucumber sensitive mask

Even ultra-sensitive skin likes cucumber. Depending on how thickly you apply the mask, any left over keeps for a day or two in the fridge.

10g (¹/₂oz) brewer's yeast (or grind up brewer's yeast tablets)
10g (¹/₂oz) finely powdered oats
7.5cm (3 inch) chunk of cucumber
2 tablespoons plain yogurt
1 teaspoon runny honey
1 drop rose essential oil

Mix together the yeast and oats in a small bowl and set aside. Peel the chunk of cucumber and liquidise it in a food processor or herb grinder until it's – literally – liquid. Add the yogurt and honey then whizz again for a few seconds, to mix. Add the brewer's yeast and the oats to the cucumber/honey mixture, drop in the rose essential oil, and whizz yet again until smooth. Apply to a cleansed face and skin, and leave on for 20–30 minutes. Remove either with a muslin washcloth dunked in warm water, or by splashing with water. Follow with a light spritz of rosewater, if you choose, and moisturiser.

Sensitive skins also love... Gentle, soothing
herbs like comfrey, chamomile and rose. Steer clear of
stimulating herbs (lavender, mint, nettle, sage, southernwood,
thyme and rosemary), avoid products containing alcohol, and be
aware that many essential oils can trigger sensitivity if you're
vulnerable. Meanwhile, sensitive skins – like all skin types –
should do a patch test (see page 145) before trying new skin
concoctions, and watch for any reactions before using the
product on face or body.

CUCUMBER
Cucumis sativus

As long ago as 1653 cucumber's role to cleanse and cool the face was chronicled by herbalist Culpeper, who added: 'it's also excellent for sun-burning, freckles and morphew' (a rather unsexy name for scurf, or scaly skin). Peeled and juiced, cucumber makes a lovely hot-weather skin lotion – on its own, or 50/50 with rosewater. It has a soothing, softening action in lotions and creams, while helping to de-clog pores; moosh with yogurt (or use the recipe here), as a face pack. Slices make the quickest and simplest of eye masks, with a blissfully soothing and slightly de-puffing action.

You can readily buy cucumbers, of course. Originally from the tropics, they're also fun to grow in a greenhouse or hot spot in the garden (though very thirsty). After a slow start, they become so prolific you'll find you have enough cucumbers to make face lotion for your friends, family (if not your entire town) – so I like to pickle them, too. Mmmmm...

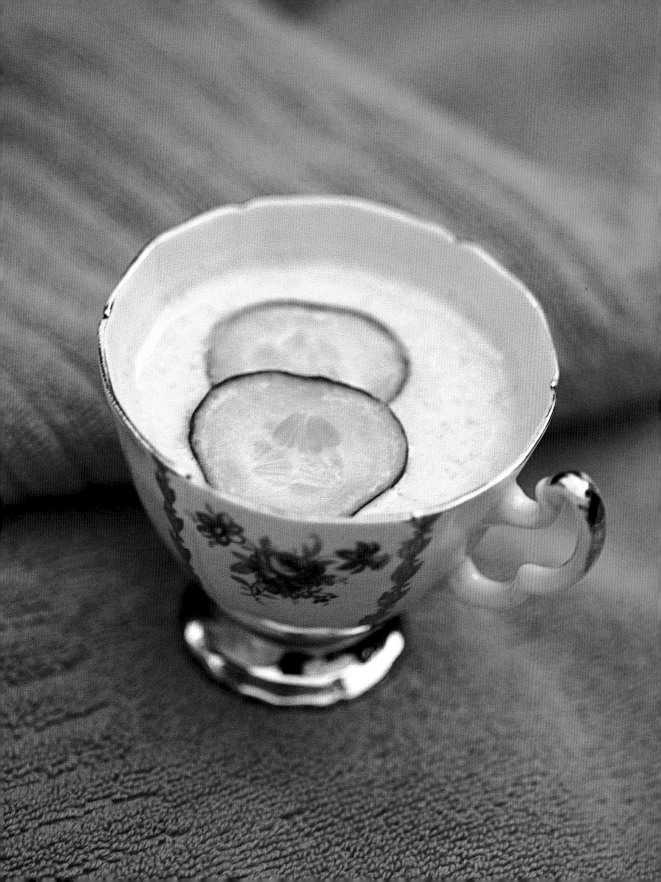

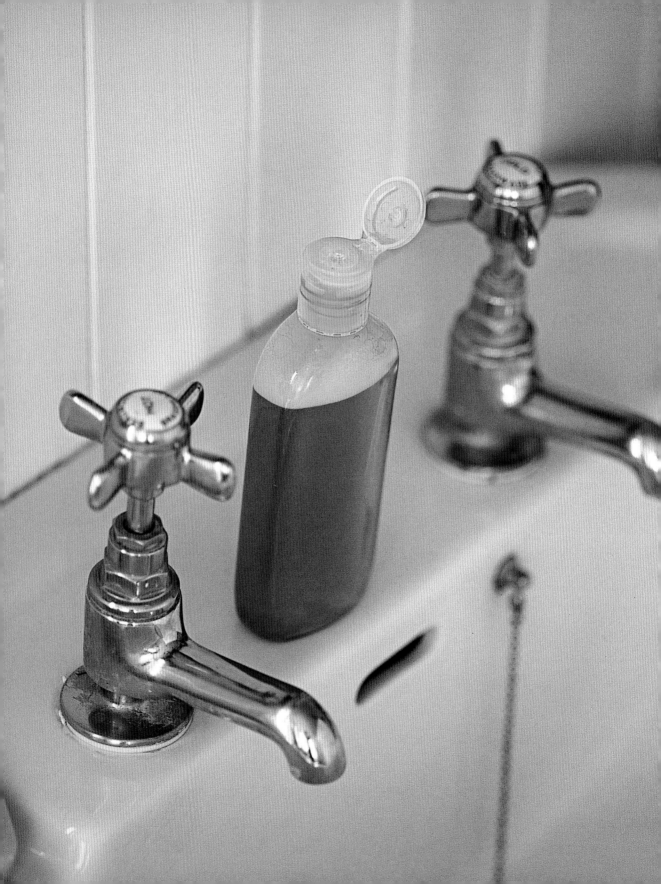

foaming herbal facewash

Soapwort is a very lightly foaming natural cleanser which – unlike most commercial facewashes – won't strip your skin. That helps to maintain skin's natural balance. It's great for a feeling of freshness from a little lather – don't expect a mass of bubbles!

50g (2oz) fresh soapwort root or
  25g (1oz) dried soapwort
50g (2oz) fresh chopped herbs or
  25g (1oz) dried herbs – a mixture of mint
  (invigorating), sage and rosemary (both antiseptic)
  would be perfect
1 litre (1³/4 pints) filtered, mineral or rainwater

Scrub and peel the freshly harvested soapwort root (soaking it for 1 hour before peeling makes the task easier – and I swear by my rubber-handled GoodGrips potato peeler). Put the root or dried soapwort in a pan with the herbs, pour over the water and cover. Bring to the boil and simmer for 10 minutes. Remove from the heat and allow to cool thoroughly; then strain through muslin and bottle the liquid (ideally into a bottle with a pump-action). Squirt a couple of dollops into the palm of your hands, morning and night, and massage into a dampened face. Rinse well. Use up within 1 month.

gentle cress and oatmeal skin-buffers

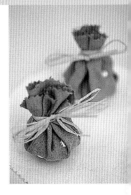

The watercress in this recipe is packed with antioxidant vitamins A and C, as well as being highly antiseptic and antibiotic. The oatmeal, meanwhile, has a skin-soothing effect, so both ingredients are very good news for problem skins.

Small bunch of watercress leaves and stalks
50ml (2fl oz) plain yogurt
60g (2¹/2oz) coarsely ground oatmeal
4 x 15 cm (6 inch) squares of muslin

Purée the cress and the yogurt in a blender. Pour the oatmeal into a bowl, add the purée and mix well. Pile 2 tablespoons of the mixture in the centre of each piece of cloth, gather up the fabric and secure round the mixture with a length of string, ribbon or raffia. Put the skin-buffing bags in a plastic bag in the fridge, where they'll keep for a few days. After cleansing at night, moisten your face with water and dampen the chilled bag. Massage any oily or blemished zones with the dampened cress bag, squeezing it gently to release the extracts. Leave your skin to dry naturally.

TIP

Most toners for oily skins work by stripping skin. My advice is to go gently, so skin can actually rebalance itself. For a gentle toner, make a tea of 2 tablespoons dried chamomile and 1 tablespoon dried rosemary poured over 225ml (8fl oz) boiling water. Strain out the herbs and keep the bottle in the fridge. Applied to cleansed skin on a pad of cotton wool, it gently tones and soothes. My bet is that your skin will soon settle down.

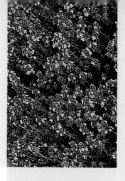

peppermint and thyme facial steam

Lots of problem-skin sufferers feel the need to steam skin occasionally – and mint and thyme are the perfect herbs to use, because they are highly effective antibacterials, helping to purify the complexion. Facial steaming is the best way to superclean your skin pore-deep, ridding it of city grime or dirt, as it encourages pores to expel toxins. However, it should be avoided by anyone with a tendency to broken veins.

2 handfuls of fresh mint leaves or 1 tablespoon dried mint
1 teaspoon fresh thyme leaves or $^1/_2$ teaspoon dried thyme leaves
600ml (1 pint) filtered, mineral or rainwater
2 drops peppermint essential oil (optional)

Place the herbs in a pan and add the water, then bring to the boil. Remove from the stove and add the essential oil. Allow to cool slightly, then pour into a bowl set on a low table. Lean over the bowl and cover your head with a thick towel, making sure the sides of the bowl are enclosed. The steam will open the pores and cause you to perspire, helping to release the trapped toxins and debris from the skin; the mint will have an antiseptic effect. Do this once or twice a week, whichever you prefer. (It's a good idea to steam before you use a mask, to increase the mask's effectiveness.)

TIP

Mix a handful of thyme with an equal quantity of dried lavender and comfrey and infuse in a jugful of hot water. When cooled, use as a shine-boosting hair rinse.

THYME
Thymus vulgaris

The heady scent of thyme can evoke the warmth of summer even when it's blowing a gale outside. It's a phenomenal bug-buster and encourages the flow of blood to the surface of the skin. Used in beautycare, thyme's good for problem skins (which need to be kept scrupulously clean), for any kind of stimulating facial tonic and as a soap ingredient. If a beauty recipe calls for honey, meanwhile, try using 'thyme honey' – harvested from thyme-frequenting bees, which is especially soothing and healing. Thyme is highly effective in deodorants – and, like rosemary, helps to keep hair soft, silky and free of dandruff. Thyme works on the senses, too: just a breath can help sharpen the mind and stimulate memory, while calming nerves. (Making it perfect to add to your bath, for times when you need to think clearly or pep yourself up.) Compact and bushy, thyme comes in many different varieties but it's common thyme that you'll want in your beauty arsenal. Unlike many aromatic herbs, thyme is happiest in deep, rich soil, where its pretty lavender-coloured flowers will attract bees to the garden.

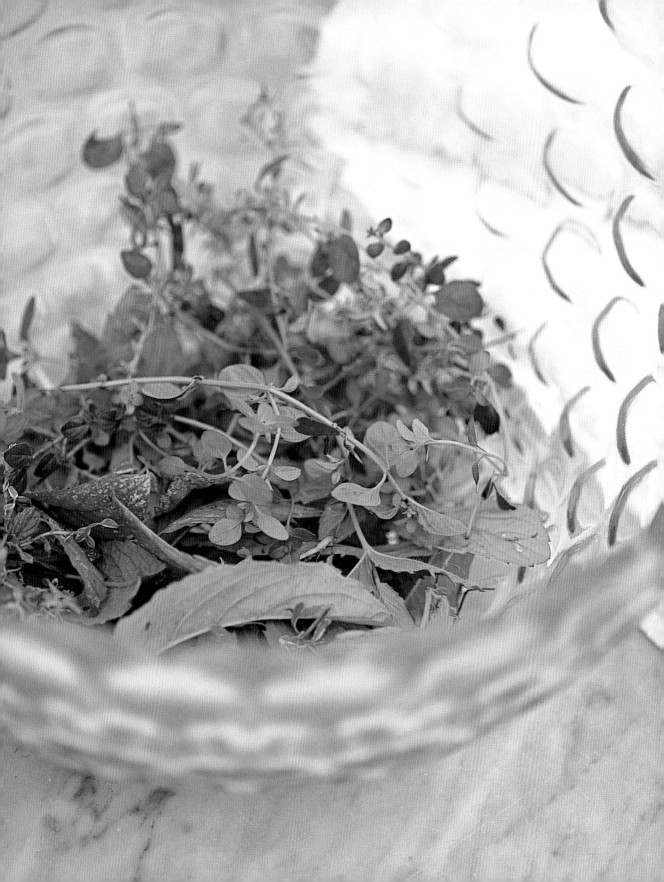

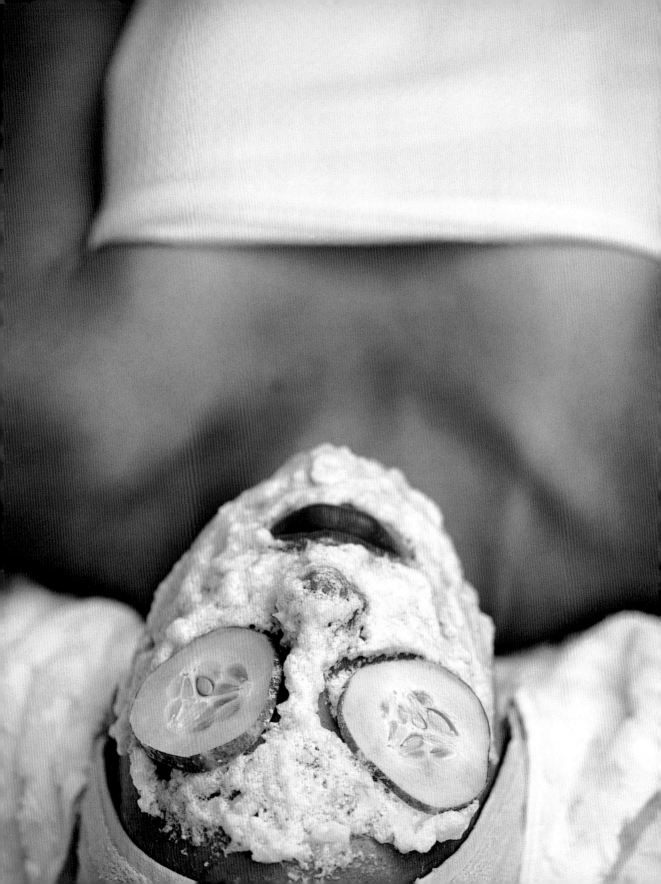

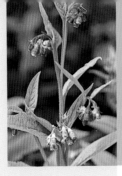

COMFREY
Symphytum officinale

Comfrey makes skin go 'Aaaaah…': it's fantastically soothing and healing, with elements that bind tissues and stimulate new cell growth. The magic skin-calming ingredient is allantoin (which you'll often find listed on ingredients labels, though the cosmetic industry often relies on a synthetic 'copy' of this beauty wonder-plant). Ninon de L'Enclos, a legendary seventeenth-century French beauty, is alleged to have used comfrey (among other herbs) to keep her skin lovely. And it's not only for skin: comfrey has been known for centuries as 'knitbone', because it can help repair fractures. (The Romans called it *conferva* – join together – hence 'comfrey'.) Herbalists use it for eczema and psoriasis. The leaves and root (fresh or dried) are the useful bits of the plant, though the short-lived flowers are very pretty. Comfrey is an amazingly balanced herb – both astringent and emollient, seeming to adapt to what individual skin needs; use it in lotions, creams or balms for oily, problem and dry complexions (while hands just adore it). As for growing comfrey? Even a small clump will soon bulk up into a strong, healthy plant when tucked into a dampish spot. Organic gardeners – like me – swear by it; the leaves can be steeped in water to make a somewhat antisocial stinky tea that acts like a miraculous plant food, when watered on. (Be aware, though, that Russian comfrey – a close relation – is considered by some to be a skin irritant.)

comfrey acne mask

50g (2oz) fresh comfrey leaves and flowers (if in season) or
  25 g (1 oz) dried comfrey
225 m (8fl oz) freshly boiled filtered, mineral or rainwater
1 egg white
50g (2 oz) Fuller's earth

Put the comfrey in a bowl and pour the boiling water over it. Cover and allow to cool completely, then strain. In a second bowl, mix the egg white and the Fuller's earth and moisten with 2 tablespoons of the comfrey liquid. Apply the mask all over your face avoiding the eyes and mouth area. Leave for 20–25 minutes. To remove, soak cotton wool pads in the remaining comfrey infusion and sweep over your face until it's clean. Allow the skin to dry naturally.

cucumber anti-blemish mask

Cucumber is calming while rosemary is a super-effective antiseptic. You'll find the egg white will tauten on your face.

2.5 cm (1 inch) chunk of cucumber
1 drop rosemary essential oil
1 egg white

Whizz the cucumber in a blender until it becomes completely liquid, then add the drop of rosemary essential oil. Whisk the egg white until stiff, fold in the cucumber mixture and smooth over the face avoiding the eyes and mouth area. Remove after 15 minutes using a clean, damp washcloth.

TIP

If you have a spotty back or shoulders, ask a friend or partner to apply the mixture to your back: it makes a wonderful 'back pack'.

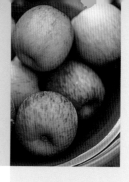

apple zit blaster

Just the thing if you feel a pimple forming, and it couldn't be simpler. Pour boiling water over a slice of apple and wait a few minutes until it becomes soft. Remove from the water, wait until it's just warm, then place on the pimple. Leave in place for 20 minutes, then peel off and sweep the area lightly with a moistened cotton wool pad.

apple toning treatment

Use this treatment at least once a week and you should see an improvement in acne, break-outs, even boils. Cut one apple into chunks, put in a blender and whizz to a pulpy juice. Lie down, put a band over your hair-line and smooth the pulp over your face avoiding the eyes and mouth area. Relax for 15–20 minutes. Rinse thoroughly and apply a light moisturiser everywhere except the T-zone.

willow blemish buster

The salicylic acid in willow leaves is what dries out spots effectively.

10g (¹/₂oz) fresh willow leaves
50ml (2fl oz) cider vinegar

Chop the willow leaves and pour the vinegar over them. Pour into a bottle and shake well, then refrigerate. Shake every day for a week, then strain off the vinegar into a sterilised bottle. Apply the liquid with a cotton wool pad to pimples.

APPLE
Malus species

An apple a day certainly keeps the skin doctor away… Apple is highly antiseptic, protecting skin from infection and killing bacteria, while being rich in minerals and vitamins A and C. Malic acid – which gives apples their tartness – is a natural alpha-hydroxy acid which gently exfoliates, smoothes and brightens dull complexions. (No wonder apples have been part of home-grown beauty regimes since – well, probably since Eve and the Garden of Eden…) Many germs are unable to survive in apple juice. The double-whammy? Eat an apple and its prized fibre-rich pectin will have skin-soothing, restorative properties.

As for growing apples? Even small gardens have room for these prettily flowering, generously fruiting trees, now that they're available as down-sized 'Minarette' or 'Ballerina' trees, which can even be grown in pots.

TIP

If you have a habit of touching your face – and many sufferers of spots or problem skins do – then try to break the habit. And if you can't, become a bit obsessive about washing your hands, as it's so easy to transfer germs to your complexion, which in turn can cause spots to become infected.

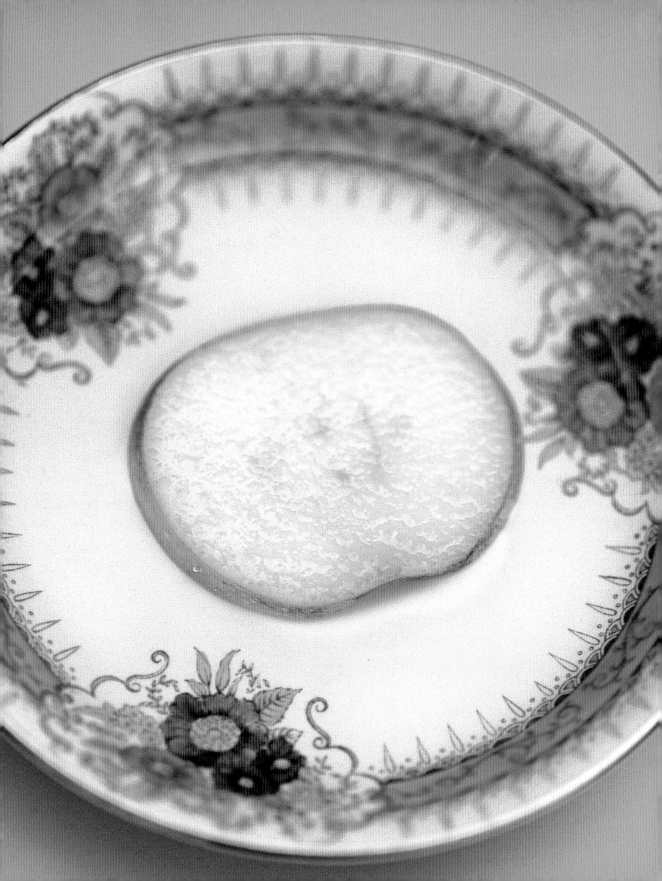

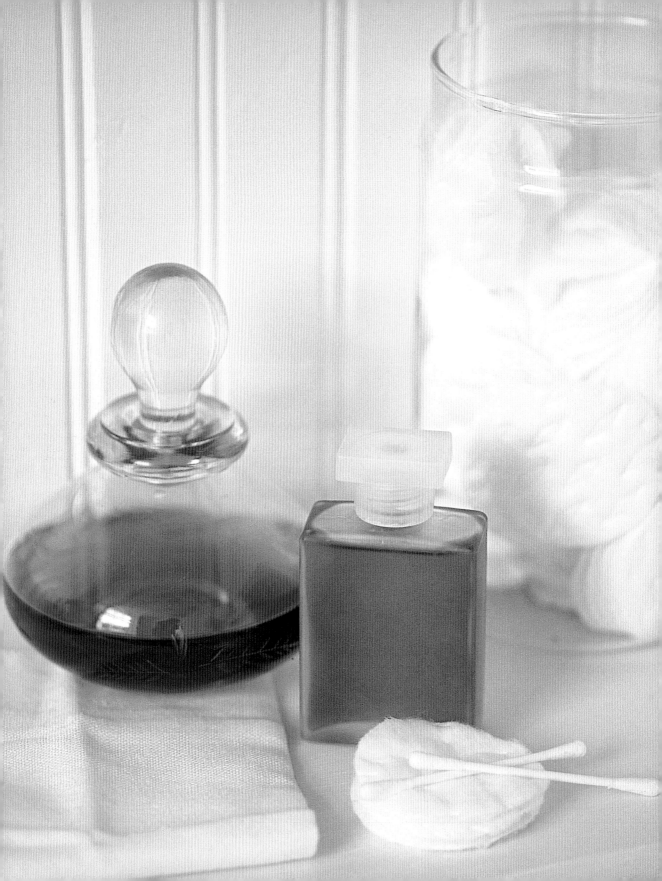

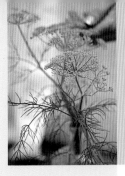

FENNEL
Foeniculum vulgare

This is gorgeous, gorgeous, gorgeous, when grown in the garden. (And the umbrella-like flowers of bronze fennel – *Foeniculum purpureum* – are among my favourite for flower arranging.) The bulbs of Florence fennel, meanwhile – the sort you find at the vegetable counter – can be zooshed into cooling, soothing face masks; you can also make a soothing eye compress by drenching cotton wool pads in a tea made from the seeds of any type of fennel.

Want to try growing your own? Like many herbs, fennel is delightfully low-maintenance: it likes a sunny spot and to be left Garbo-ishly alone. (The bulb-producing edible sweet fennel likes plenty of water, however, to bulk up.) Oh, and one last thing: fennel's said to be the herb of immortality, associated with ageing well and longevity. (So you might want to drink some of that fennel tea, while you're at it.)

TIP

If you're too impatient to infuse your own marigold flowers, the Neal's Yard Remedies range includes a calendula oil – and the infusing is done for you.

marigold and frankincense nourishing cleansing oil

Marigolds are one of skin's best friends, while frankincense has been renowned for its anti-ageing power since the time of the Egyptians, who used it in mummification! This blend melts make-up like magic, while the oils (which are rich in essential fatty acids) 'feed' the skin.

50g (2oz) dried marigold (calendula) flowers
50ml (2fl oz) sunflower oil
2 tablespoons hempseed oil
2 tablespoons apricot kernel oil
15 drops frankincense or rose essential oil (optional)

Place the marigold flowers in the bottom of a wide-necked glass jar and pour the sunflower oil over them. Seal and stand in a sunny window for 3 weeks, then strain off the oil. Add the hempseed and apricot kernel oils and decant into a screw-top glass bottle. If you're using the essential oil, add it drop by drop. Apply the oil from the bottle onto cotton wool pads and sweep over your complexion.

fennel and honey freshener

Honey and fennel are both reputed to have anti-ageing powers, and this light freshener is perfect if you like your face to feel really clean but not at all 'tight' after cleansing with oil-based cleanser.

50ml (2fl oz) rosewater or orange flower water
10g (1/2oz) fennel seeds
1 teaspoon runny honey

Make an infusion of the fennel seeds with the rosewater (see p. 153), and allow to sit for 24 hours before filtering through a muslin cloth or kitchen paper. Apply as a spritz or on a cotton wool pad.

grape flesh face firmer

The natural exfoliants and antioxidants contained in grapes leave skin feeling ultra-silky but firm, while the fruit acids have a lightly exfoliating effect, brightening skin.

4 large grapes or 8 smaller grapes

Split and skin the grapes and remove the pips. Mash the flesh to a pulp and apply to the skin avoiding the eyes and mouth area. Leave for 10–15 minutes. This feels slimy as it glides onto skin, but you'll find it refreshingly cool and tingly, too. Rinse off with warm water, pat dry and moisturise as usual.

TIP

Mature skin often has a legacy of sun damage to the *décolletage*. It's said that an infusion (see p. 153) of elderflower can help keep the skin white, as well as protect it from the effects of the sun. (Although of course, you should always apply sun protection to this vulnerable zone, too.) At night, follow with a few drops of sweet almond oil massaged into the area – or use the Madonna Lily Neck Treatment, p. 53.

lettuce softening tonic

Lettuce has an amazing skin-softening effect. This is good after cleansing or any time your skin is feeling hot and bothered or parched.

300ml (1/2 pint) water (preferably rainwater) or use rosewater (or 50/50)
1 head of lettuce (any variety), chopped

Heat the liquid until almost boiling. Pour over the chopped lettuce and steep for a few hours. Strain the liquid through a sieve and pour into a sterilised bottle and seal. Apply using a cotton wool pad.

Mature skins also love facial massage... Massage nourishes the skin with blood and drains away the lymph that leads to puffiness, and for me, just 5 minutes spent on facial massage is the fastest way to take off 5 years when I feel (and look) tired. I've outlined a technique on p. 136.

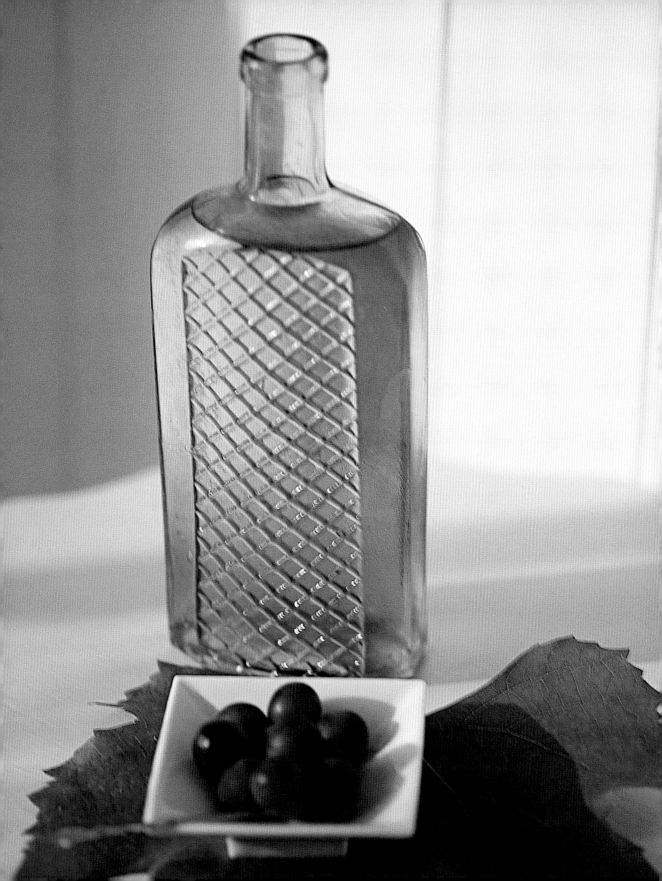

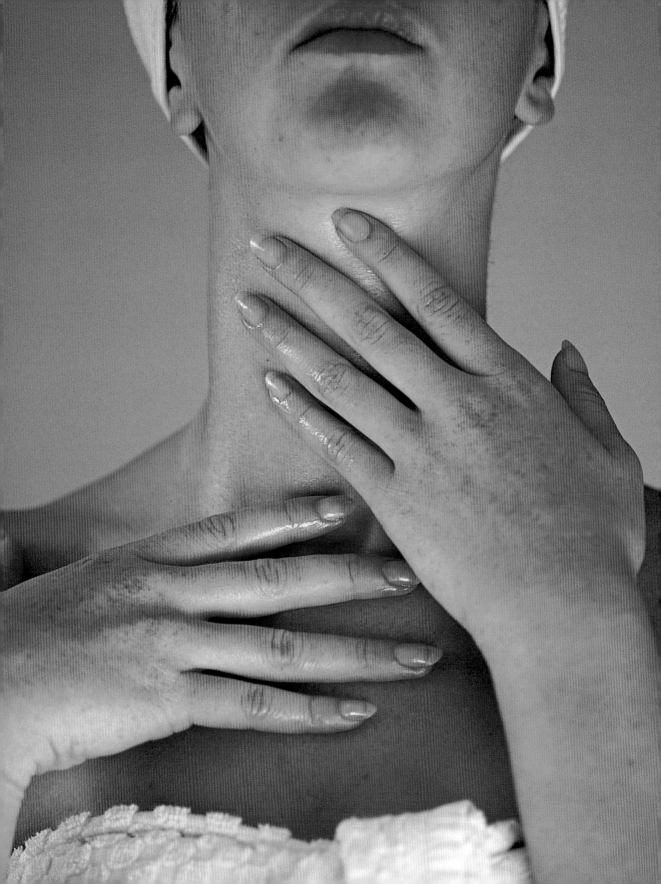

vitamin-boost moisturiser

Some women swear by piercing a capsule of vitamin E and simply smearing the contents over their face. This recipe, however, turbo-charges the effect of the vitamin E with borage flower (starflower) oil, in a gorgeously moisturising blend that's one of my favourites in the book.

1 tablespoon fresh marigold (calendula) *petals or*
   1 teaspoon dried marigold flowers
150ml (¹/4 pint) water
20g (³/4oz) beeswax
100ml (3¹/2 fl oz) extra virgin olive oil
1 tablespoon vegetable glycerine
30ml (1fl oz) wheatgerm oil
2 capsules starflower oil
2 capsules vitamin E oil
15 drops frankincense essential oil

Put the herb and the water in a saucepan and bring to the boil to make a decoction (see p. 153). Leave to cool, then strain. Heat the beeswax in the oil in the top of a double-boiler until melted (see p. 153). Remove from the heat and slowly add the glycerine and 2 tablespoons of the herbal decoction, beating well with a hand-whisk or an electric whisk. Pierce the capsules to extract the starflower and vitamin E oils, then beat in these and the wheatgerm oil. Transfer into a sterilised pot or jar and cover when completely cold. Use within 2 months.

madonna lily neck treatment

It might seem extravagant to use lily bulbs – but have you seen the price of neck creams lately? If you grow Madonna lilies, the bulbs should ideally be lifted straight from the ground, so they will be plump and juicy; scrub thoroughly to remove any earth. If you use a bulb that you buy from a garden centre, the skin may have toughened and you may need to peel it.

1 Madonna lily (Lilium candidum) *bulb*
50ml (2fl oz) rosewater
50g (2 oz) beeswax
2 tablespoons apricot kernel oil
¹/2 teaspoon vitamin E oil
1 teaspoon runny honey
4 drops grapefruit seed extract

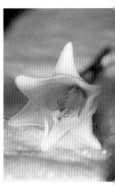

Use half a dozen 'scales' from the lily; peel or clean them and place in a blender with the rosewater, then zoosh until the mixture is frothy and smooth. Strain it into the top of a double-boiler (see p. 153) and heat for 5 minutes. Pour into a jug or bowl and set aside. Heat the beeswax in the oils in the top of the double-boiler until melted. Stir in the honey and the 'lily juice'; you may want to use a hand-blender for smoothness. Add the grapefruit seed extract drop by drop. Pour into a sterilised jar and allow to set firm. Use nightly, massaged into the neck using upward strokes.

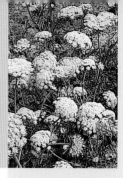

vita-carrot mask

Carrot is incredibly rich in vitamin A, which has an anti-ageing activity when applied topically to the skin. This is good for even the most sensitive skins.

1 large carrot
1 tablespoon sweet almond oil
5 drops jasmine essential oil (optional)

Peel and liquidise the carrot and strain off the juice (and you can drink this!) Blend the pulp with the sweet almond oil and add the jasmine essential oil, if using, drop by drop. (I also like to add a few jasmine flowers, when they're in season.) Lie on an old – or not very special! – towel and apply the pulp to your cleansed face avoiding the eyes and mouth area. Relax and allow the mask to work for 10–15 minutes. Rinse well with warm water, then pat dry and moisturise as usual.

Mature skins also love... Comfrey,
chamomile, jasmine, honey,
evening primrose oil, marigold,
olive oil, wheatgerm oil...

CARROT
Daucus carota

Your mother probably told you to eat up your carrots. Well, she should really have been telling you to slather them on your skin, too: carrots are packed with skin-renewing vitamins including provitamins A, B and C. (Which makes them useful for ageing skins, because they help restore skin's elasticity, helping make it touch-me-soft; they also have a tautening, 'face-lifting' action – as well as being anti-inflammatory and helping to fight off skin infections.)

Carrots aren't a breeze to grow: they like a sandy, free-draining soil, otherwise they create some very interesting shapes through 'fanging', and you'll often hear allotmenteers bleating about carrot root fly. (Which can actually be avoided by covering with fleece.) There's a form of wild carrot that can be harvested, too: *Daucus sylvestris*, often found growing at the edge of woodland or fields, and by the roadside. For flavour, nothing beats a freshly pulled carrot. And in beauty terms, the fresher the better, as the vitamin content dwindles when they're stored for a long time. But if you'd rather buy your carrots, make sure they're organic: in the UK, even the government advises peeling carrots before eating, because of the high levels of pesticide residues that have been measured in samples. Oh, and if you're trying to quit your Starbucks caffeine habit, the seeds of carrot make a pleasant afternoon tea.

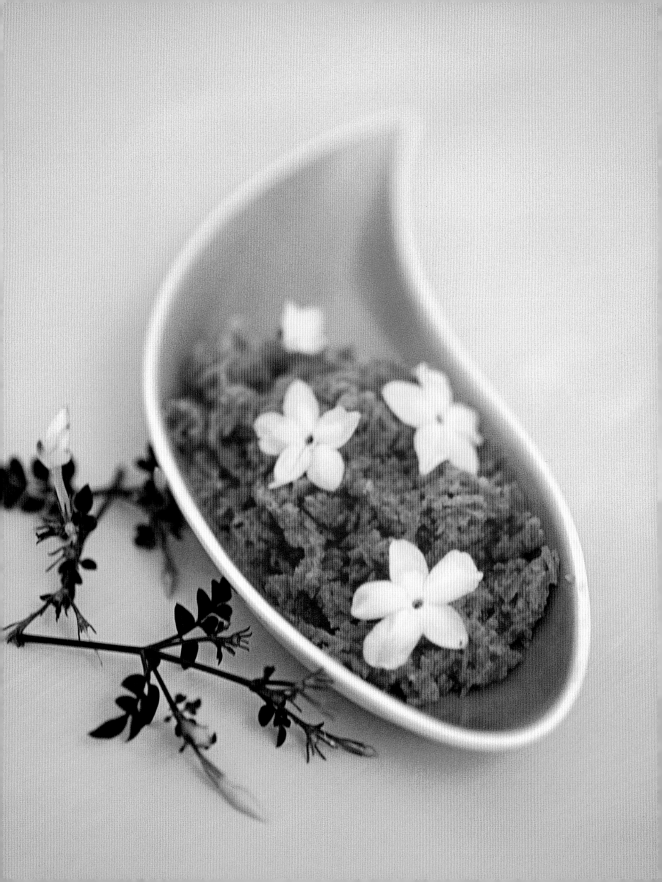

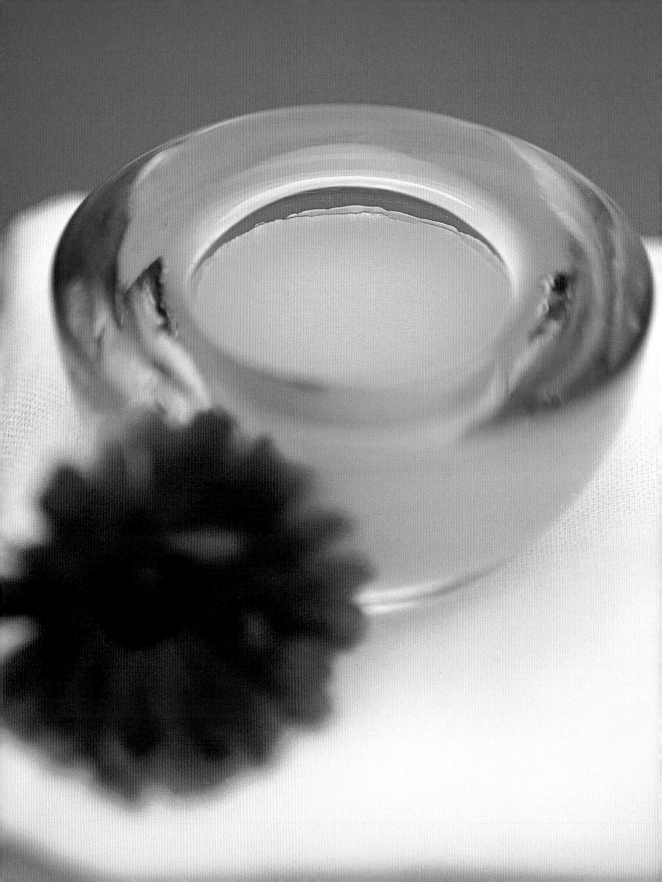

skin S.O.S. essentials

I like to have the following to hand for beauty (and health) emergencies:

• An aloe vera plant growing on a sunny windowsill in the kitchen, to slice off to treat minor cooking burns and scalds

• Arnica cream (for bruises)

• Honey is excellent as a skin S.O.S. It's naturally antiseptic, can be applied to cuts and grazes – or literally smeared on lips as a lip-healer. (Try to resist the temptation to lick it straight off again!)

• Lavender essential oil – one of the few essential oils that can be applied direct to the skin and a miracle worker for minor burns

• Rescue Remedy (this one's an absolute must for stressful times – and remember: stress shows up on your face, fast...)

• Tea tree essential oil – great for cuts, grazes (and outbreaks of athlete's foot)

all-purpose calendula skin salve

I keep this balm in the first-aid cupboard for all sorts of beauty emergencies: rashes, itching, sore spots, inflammations and flakiness. (If you can't get hold of marigold flowers, the Neal's Yard Remedies calendula-infused oil is a perfect base for this product.)

25g (1oz) dried marigold (calendula) flowers
150ml (1/4 pint) sunflower oil
25g (1oz) beeswax, grated

Place the marigold flowers in the bottom of a wide-necked glass jar. Pour on the oil, and leave the mixture to steep on a windowsill. (Make sure there's no air trapped and that the flowers are well covered.) Shake daily for about 3 weeks, by which time you'll have a wonderful soothing oil base for the salve. Strain through a fine cloth into a bowl, squeezing and pressing the flowers until the last drops are filtered.

To make the salve itself, heat the oil with the beeswax in the top of a double-boiler (see p. 153) and stir until thoroughly melted using a chopstick or spoon. To test the consistency, drop a small amount of the salve mixture onto a saucer, and put it in the freezer for 1 minute to cool. If you want a harder salve, reheat and add a little more beeswax. If you feel the salve is too hard, reheat and add a little extra oil. (The weather makes a difference, too, so you may need more beeswax when it's warm outside.) Pour the salve into a wide-necked jar and allow to cool and solidify. Store away from heat and light.

gentle eye make-up remover oil

This oil-based make-up remover, infused with gentle, soothing plant goodness, will not dry out the delicate tissue around the eyes.

10g (¹/₂oz) dried marigold (calendula) flowers
1 teaspoon dried eyebright
2 tablespoons olive oil
2 tablespoons avocado oil
2 tablespoons sunflower oil

Put the dried herbs in a wide-necked jar and cover with the oils making sure the herbs are fully submerged. Seal then leave for about 4 weeks on a windowsill. After the required time, strain then strain again, either through kitchen paper or muslin, and pour into a dry, sterilised bottle with a screwtop or a cork, or a bottle with a drop dispenser. To use the infused oil, put just 3–4 drops of the oil onto a wetted cotton wool pad that you've squeezed to get rid of excess moisture. Sweep the cotton wool pad across the eye area, but avoid getting the formula into your eyes. Be absolutely sure to use a clean pad for each eye.

   (If you want a shortcut, you can 'cook' the dried herbs in the oil in a double-boiler (see p. 153) for 15 minutes, rather than waiting for sunlight and time to infuse their goodness into the oil. Cool thoroughly, strain then strain again before transferring to a sterilised bottle.)

cucumber refreshing gel

The cooling effect of cucumber with aloe vera is utterly soothing and restorative.

2.5 cm (1 inch) slice aloe vera leaf or
   1 tablespoon aloe vera gel, available from a
   natural foodstore
2.5 cm (1 inch) chunk cucumber
¹/₄ teaspoon cornflour
1 tablespoon witch hazel
1 drop grapefruit seed extract

Pound the peeled aloe vera leaf or the aloe gel with the cucumber in a pestle and mortar (or whizz in a herb grinder) until they are smoothly blended. Then put in a double-boiler (see p. 153) with the cornflour and heat until almost boiling. Allow to cool slightly then add the witch hazel and the grapefruit seed extract. Pour into a small, sterile glass jar and put in the fridge to cool completely. Lightly dab the gel onto the 'orbital bone' around the eye (essentially, the eye socket area).

Be super-aware that natural cosmetics – made without synthetic preservatives – can become contaminated: immediately ditch any eye preparation if it starts to smell different or if you get any kind of eye infection. Always ensure your hands are clean when you use any home-made eye treat. Never put a home-made infusion directly into your eyes; it may not be sufficiently sterile.

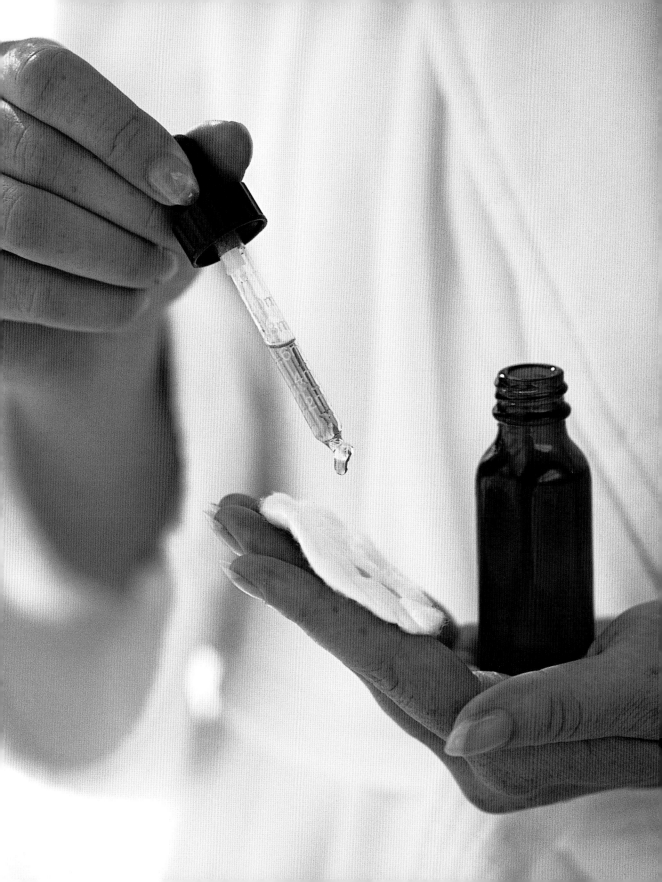

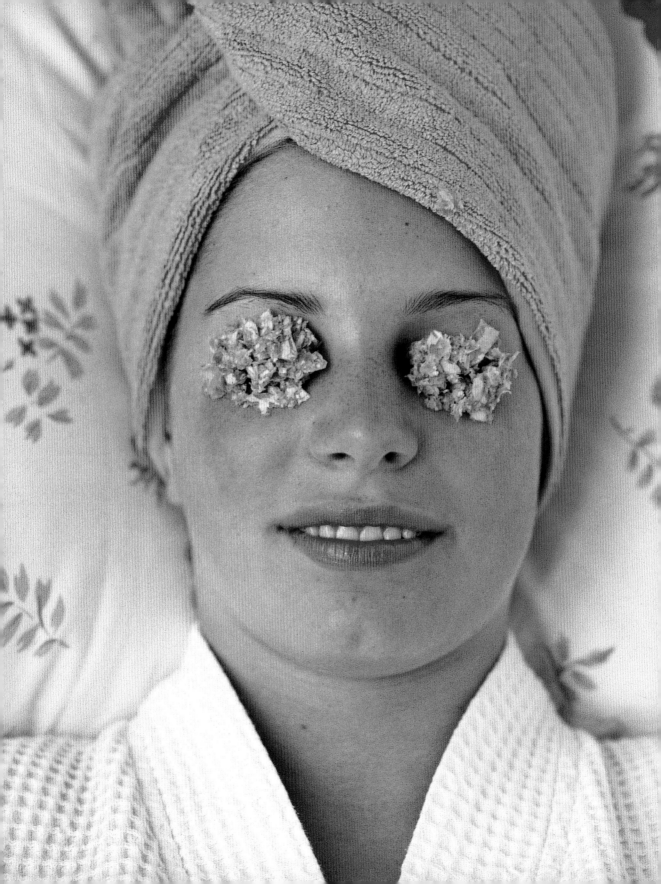

chamomile eye bag blitzer

Chamomile has a miraculous effect on tired or puffy eyes. If you know you're heading for a morning-after-the-night-before, make this infusion before you go out and it'll be ice-cold and ready for bag-blitzing, next day. (It keeps for just a few days in the fridge.) At a pinch you can also use a cold chamomile tea bag: stew in water and cool in the fridge before use.

10g (¹/₂oz) dried chamomile flowers
Freshly boiled filtered, mineral or rainwater

Place the flowers in a mug and fill with boiling water; allow to cool, strain into a sterilised jar and put in the fridge. Soak cotton wool pads in the cold tea, squeeze out the excess, and place over the eyes for 15–20 minutes. (Pads not balls, because they cover more of the eye zone.) Tap with your fingertips along the orbital bone to help the de-puffing action.

potato de-bagger

Potato has a decongesting action which works to reduce puffiness. Rather than a couple of thick slices (which is the traditional advice), I've found that thin slices are much more effective because they're in contact with the skin.

Simply slice ¹/₄ raw potato into 5–10 very thin slices that can easily be moulded to the skin. Spritz the eye area with filtered water and arrange the potato slices around the eyes. Leave in place for 10–15 minutes – and see that puffiness disappear.

rosepetal eye reviver

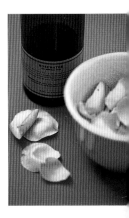

It's vital to use unsprayed rose petals, as these will be right next to your eyes. Avoid commercially grown roses as these are always drenched in pesticides. (You can use dried rose petals for this eye treat – but again, do make sure they're organic.)

Rose petals (unsprayed)
Few drops of rosewater

Pound the rose petals in a pestle and mortar adding the rosewater drop by drop until you have a mask-like, not-too-runny consistency. Lie down somewhere peaceful and scoop a small handful of the pounded roses onto each closed eye; pat into place. Relax and dream for 15–20 minutes, then swish the roses away with water. Your eyes will feel calmer and more soothed. (As an effective, de-puffing variation on this, use a few drops of cucumber juice in place of the rosewater while you pound the roses.)

TIP

If eyes are puffy in the morning, take a leaf out of supermodel Linda Evangelista's book and reach for a cube of ice. Wrap it in clingfilm and use it to 'massage away' eye bags, working in an outward direction. The cold will quickly reduce the swelling.

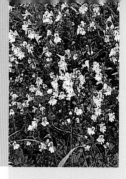

eyebright eye brightener

A quick and simple reviver for when your eyes feel tired. Stored in the fridge, this infusion will keep for 3–4 days (no longer).

10g (¹/₂oz) dried eyebright flowers
225ml (8fl oz) filtered or mineral water

Put the flowers in a pan, add the water. Bring to the boil and simmer for 5 minutes. Cool and strain, then pour into a sterilised jar. Soak 2 cotton wool pads in the mixture, squeeze to remove almost all the liquid and place the damp pads on your eyelids for 5–10 minutes.

herbal eye pillows

Try these eye pillows to help you get to sleep, during an at-home spa treatment or any time you need to relax. The weight of the grains seems to quiet the eyes – and, in turn, the mind. These make wonderful gifts, too. Your herb pillows should last for about a year; when the next lavender harvest is in, renew them.

25cm (10 inches) silky or natural fabric (cotton or linen)
150g (5oz) dried lavender flowers (or a mixture – half and half –
  of lavender and flaxseed)
6 drops lavender essential oil (optional)

Cut two rectangles of fabric, each approximately 22 x 13 cm (9 x 5¹/₂ inches). With right sides together stitch a 1cm (¹/₂ inch) seam around the two long sides and one end of the pillow, either by hand or using a sewing machine. Turn right side out. Put the flaxseed and the lavender flowers in a bowl, add the lavender essential oil, drop by drop, swirl to mix – and (using using a funnel) pour the mixture into the bag. Neatly hand-stitch the remaining end closed.

EYEBRIGHT
Euphrasia officinalis

Euphrasia is the eye-friendly herb, as its common name suggests. It grows in natural grassland and you might be able to introduce seeds of this dainty, blueish-white flowered plant into a wild, grassy corner of your garden, if you don't pamper it too much. If not, the dried herb is just as effective. Eyebright's power was recorded as long ago as the fourteenth century, when it was deemed useful for all 'evils of the eye'. The herb is rich in the mineral zinc, which helps repair skin tissues – probably explaining why it's good at caring for the fragile skin around the eyes. Eyebright is also a good skin disinfectant.

TIP

The herbal eye pillows on this page can be made of almost any natural material, but silk is particularly soothing and gentle on the skin. Vintage fabrics – like silk crêpe-de-Chine – make beautiful eye pillows: those featured here are made from old kimono fabric.

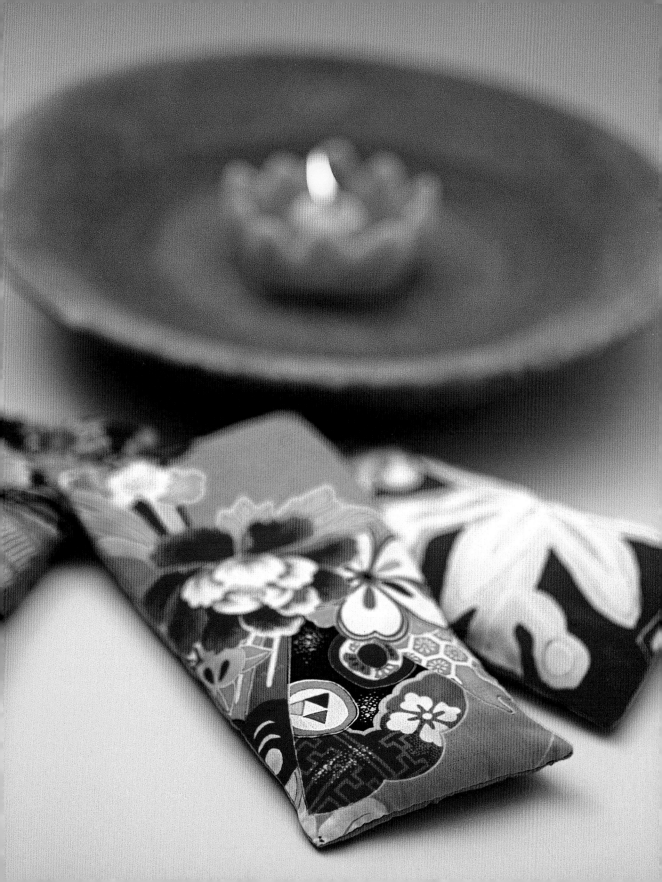

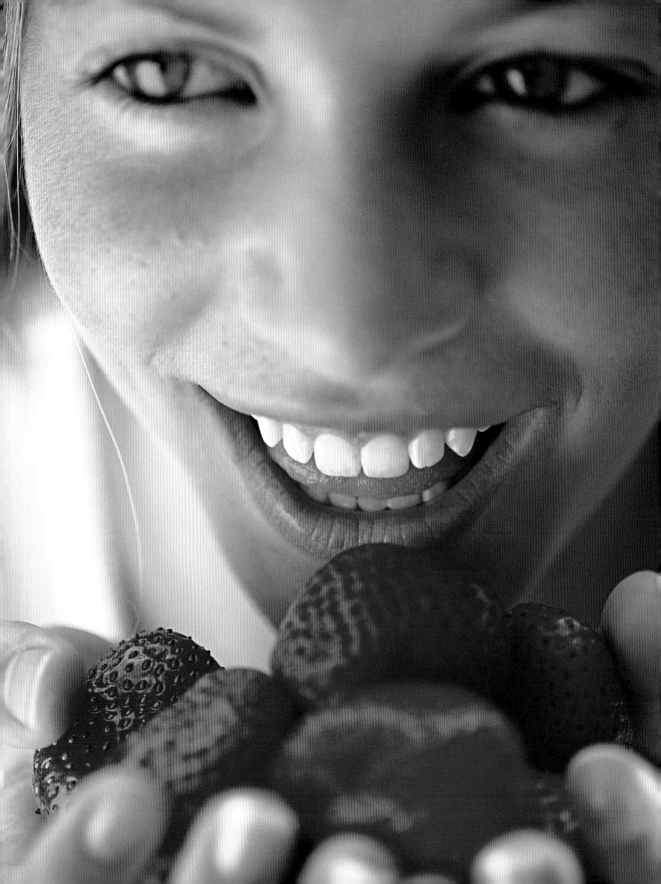

strawberry smile brightener

This is great before a special occasion; it sounds strange, but strawberries can actually lighten teeth and remove discolorations, because the malic acid has astringent properties. Of course you won't get the same effect as from a bleaching treatment done by a dentist, but your teeth will definitely look brighter and shinier.

1 ripe strawberry
$^1/_2$ teaspoon baking powder

Crush the strawberry to a pulp, then mix with the baking powder. Use a soft toothbrush to 'paint' the mixture onto teeth and allow to 'set' for 5 minutes. Then brush thoroughly to remove the mixture; rinse with plenty of water.

Teeth also love...

• Fresh sage. Rub a leaf over your teeth to make them brighter and whiter.

• Raspberries, which are reputed to help dissolve plaque when you eat them.

• Fresh spearmint. Chew on a fresh leaf to whiten the teeth, condition the gums and help prevent bad breath.

TIP

A mouthwash of calendula tea is great for healing mouth ulcers and for treating gum disease.

herbal tooth powder

Baking soda (bicarbonate of soda) is well known as a tooth cleaner and you can easily make your own, herb-flavoured powder. I prefer this to manufactured toothpastes which contain saccharin and other artificial flavourings.

100g (3$^1/_2$oz) kaolin powder
100g (3$^1/_2$oz) bicarbonate of soda
10g ($^1/_2$oz) dried raspberry leaf
5g ($^1/_4$oz) dried herbs (whatever you fancy, from spearmint, sage, fennel, or peppermint)
5g ($^1/_4$oz) myrrh powder
5g ($^1/_4$oz) dried yellow dock
5 drops peppermint essential oil (if you're using mint), sage essential oil (if you're using sage) or sweet fennel essential oil (likewise)

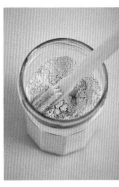

Tip the kaolin powder and the bicarbonate of soda into a mixing bowl, and pulverise the herbs in a coffee grinder or spice mill (or use a pestle and mortar). Add both the other dry ingredients and whisk together with a metal whisk, to keep air in the mixture. Add the essential oil that matches your chosen herb, and whisk again. Cover the bowl with a clean towel or dishcloth and leave it overnight. In the morning, whisk briefly again and decant into a sterilised bottle. Tap a little of the mixture onto your toothbrush morning and night, and brush as usual.

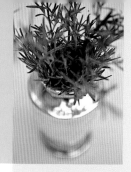

rosemary and mint mouthwash

You can use this just like any mouthwash – swig, swish, gargle – but unlike alcohol-based mouthwashes (which can dry out the inside of the mouth and actually unbalance the natural 'flora') this is gentle while still being effective. The glycerine acts as a natural sweetener.

25g (1oz) fresh rosemary or 10g (¹/₂oz) dried rosemary
25g (1oz) fresh mint or 10g (¹/₂oz) dried mint
1 litre (1³/₄ pints) boiling filtered or mineral water
30ml (1fl oz) vegetable glycerine
10–12 drops peppermint essential oil
5–10 drops myrrh essential oil

Make an infusion (see p. 153) with the herbs and the water; allow to cool and stir in the glycerine. Add the essential oils and pour into a sterilised bottle. Shake before use and discard any that remains after 2 weeks. (Don't swallow it – though it won't do you any harm if you do.)

TIP

You can also successfully freshen your breath in the following ways: chew a little fresh parsley. (This herbal garnish is rich in chlorophyll, a green plant compound that kills the bacteria that cause bad odour.) Or, chew on a dried clove, some fennel seeds or a juniper berry. Rinse your mouth with water that contains chopped watercress.

ROSEMARY
Rosmarinus officinalis

Rosemary isn't just a great breath-freshener: the herbalist Culpeper recommended rosemary 'to take away spots, marks and scars in the skin.' He was onto something: science now confirms rosemary contains an active ingredient that really does help strengthen fragile capillaries, and may even work to fade the appearance of broken veins. It's wonderfully invigorating to both skin and scalp – and acts like a jolt to the senses, delivering instant energy when strewn in a bath, or even if you brush against a bush on a sunny summer's day. (It can be a little too invigorating for some people: if you're using rosemary essential oil in a face pack, stick to 1–2 drops, as too much can be irritating.) Meanwhile, if you infuse a sprig of rosemary in hot water and drink the tea, it'll perk you up in no time. Rosemary may even be rejuvenating: readers of *Banck's Herbal* (1525) were advised to 'smell it oft and it shall keep thee youngly'.

If you're growing this herb in a pot or garden bed, remember two things: that rosemary (like many herbs) doesn't like to get its feet wet (so needs free drainage); and that it really likes a good haircut in late summer, to prevent it getting 'leggy'. If you cut back into dead rosemary wood, it won't regenerate, so make this cutting-back an annual task. I love how rosemary got its name, from the Latin for 'dew of the sea'. (That's why it's very happy by the coast.)

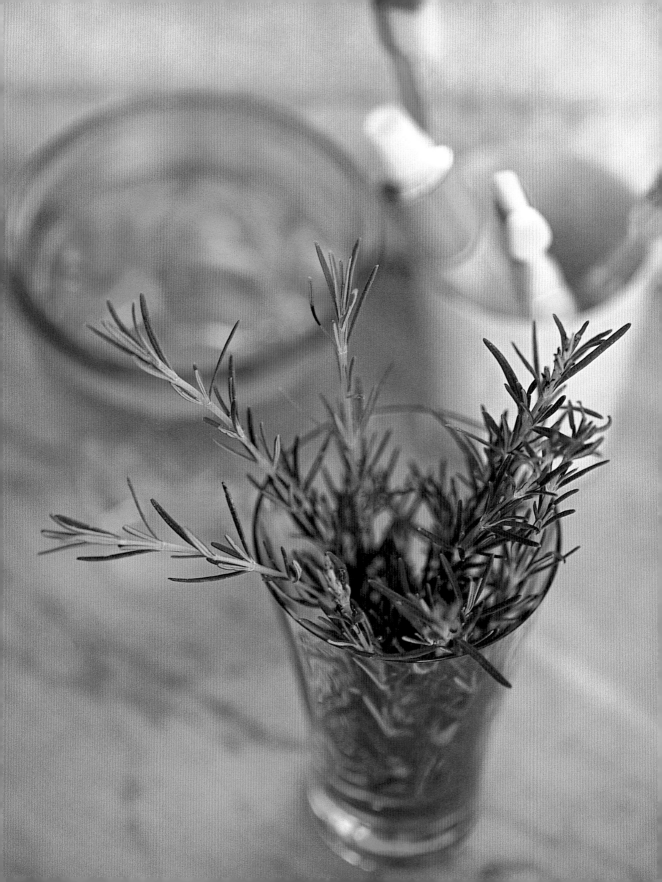

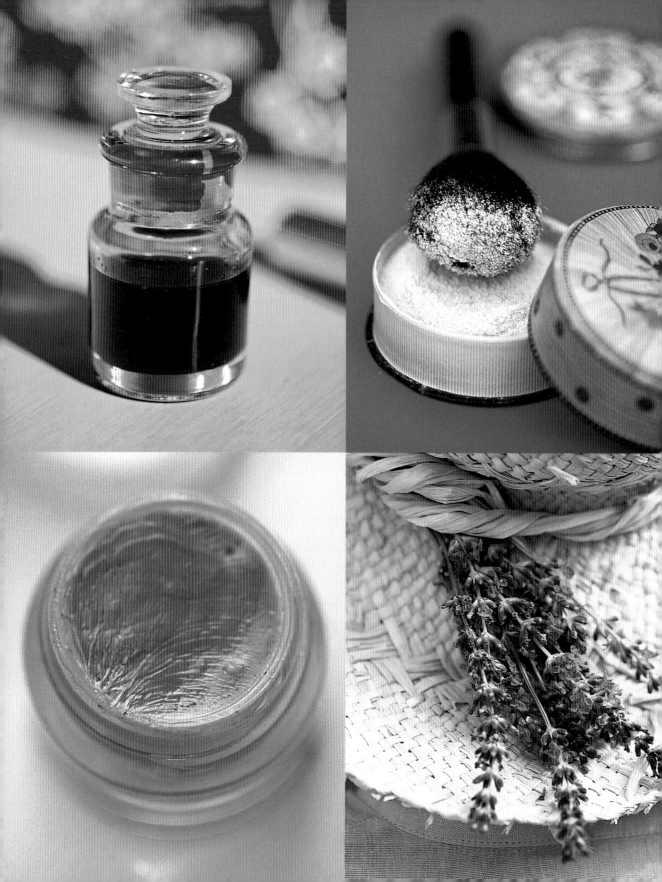

make-up

When you **take care of your skin holistically** – by which I mean eating well, breathing properly, taking exercise and exposing it to the minimum of irritants and synthetic chemicals – you should find that you need to wear **less make-up**. It's a fact: many petrochemical ingredients can block pores; **natural ingredients allow your skin to breathe and function perfectly**. So here are some alternatives to everyday make-up items – and some savvy shopping suggestions for where to find natural eyeshadows, pencils and mascaras, which are a bit of a challenge to make at home...

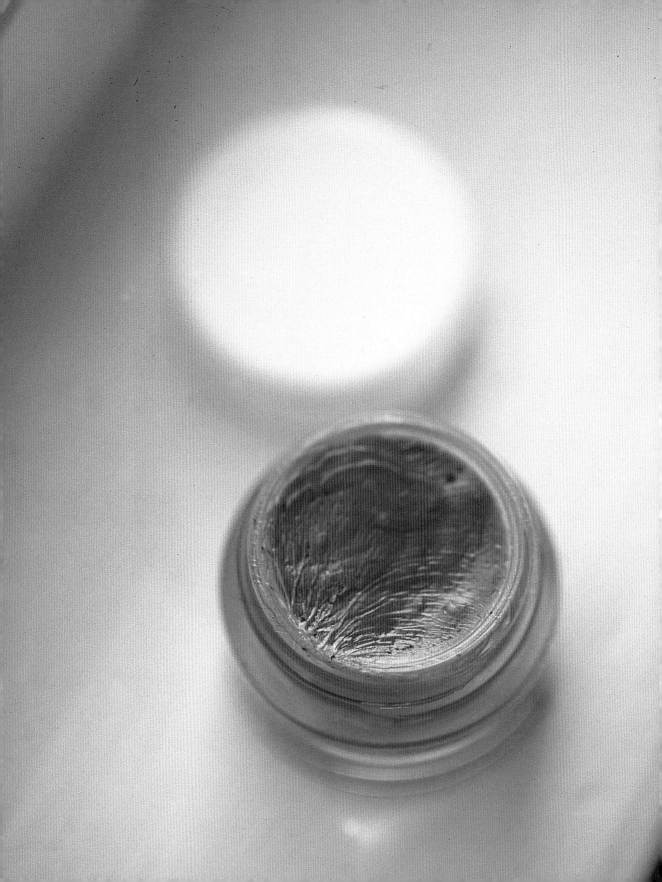

be naturally beautiful

As I've said already, when you're caring for your skin gently and naturally, you shouldn't need to wear make-up all the time. And there are some make-up items which are just impossible to make satisfactorily at home, like foundation, or natural eyeshadows and pencils. So if you feel the need to wear these – but you want to be an ultimate natural beauty – I recommend that you check out the range on offer from Aveda (who avoid petrochemical ingredients), as well as 'cult' natural brand Dr Hauschka, who offers a full make-up collection that's as natural as it gets (from foundations to lip glosses). Jane Iredale make-up is also terrific: it's based on crushed mineral pigments. My friend Leslie Kenton, for instance – one of the original natural beauty gurus – turned me on to Jane Iredale Amazing Base Loose Minerals SPF20, which whisks onto skin to conceal imperfections; it's a concealer, foundation, powder and sunscreen all in one – and I reckon lives up to its 'amazing' name! (See RESOURCES, pp. 154–7 to track down these ranges.)

glossy lip gloss

Apply to lips for instant sheen and gloss – or slick it over a (natural) lipstick, for shine with greater depth of colour.

1 teaspoon grated cocoa butter
½ teaspoon coconut oil
1 teaspoon sweet almond oil
½ teaspoon beeswax
1 teaspoon aloe vera gel (available from natural foodstores)

If the cocoa butter is solid (as it tends to be if the ambient temperature is cold), you can grate it first using a fine grater (I find a Microplane is perfect). Heat together the cocoa butter, the coconut oil, almond oil and beeswax in a double-boiler (see p. 153) until melted; remove from the heat and stir in the aloe vera gel. Whisk everything together. Pour the mixture into a small, sterilised container and allow to cool completely.

think pink lip tint

Beetroot produces a fab, strawberry-pink lip tint. I'm addicted to mine. You need to grate cooked beetroot to extract the juice (make more than you need), or use a bottled pure beetroot juice, available from natural foodstores.

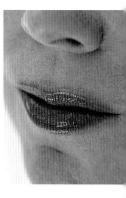

2 tablespoons sweet almond oil
10g (½oz) beeswax
1 tablespoon beetroot juice
 (or less, for a paler balm)
4 drops peppermint essential oil

Gently heat the oil and the beeswax in a double-boiler (see p. 153 for technique). Remove from heat and gradually add the beetroot juice, a teaspoon at a time, until you get the colour you like; whisk very well with a fork or small whisk. Add the peppermint essential oil, whisk again and transfer into a small sterilised pot.

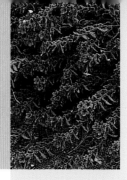

beetroot and glycerine cheek and lip tint

BeneFit Cosmetics popularised the idea of 'cheek tints': sheer, liquid colour that delivers a just-got-back-from-a-seaside-walk glow. I wanted to come up with an all-natural version – and this is it.

45g (1¹/₂oz) raw beetroot, grated
3 tablespoons vegetable glycerine

Put the beetroot and the glycerine in the top of a double-boiler (see p. 153). Heat gently for 15 minutes, cool then strain into a small jug. Pour it into a sealable container. Shake before use, then apply a dab to your cheeks, blending well. Try smooshing it on your lips, too (it tastes delicious). I like to finish with the Glossy Lip Gloss (see p. 71).

rosebud lips

This luscious lip-slick gets its purplish-pink colour from alkanet.

75ml (3fl oz) olive oil
1 tablespoon jojoba oil
45g (1¹/₂oz) dried alkanet root, chopped
20g (³/₄oz) beeswax
9 drops rose essential oil

Gently heat both oils in the top of a double-boiler (see p. 153) for about 10 minutes. Remove from the heat, add the alkanet root and steep for around 30 minutes, to extract the colour from the root. Strain the root from the oils through a muslin cloth and compost the root. Return the oils to the double-boiler with the beeswax. Once this has melted, remove from heat and add the rose essential oil, drop by drop. Pour into small, sterilised pots or jars. Allow to cool thoroughly before capping.

ALKANET
Alkanna tinctoria

Alkanet – also known as Spanish bugloss – is useful if you want to tint products such as lip balms: a reddish dye can be obtained from its thick, carrot-like roots, which should be dried before use in cosmetics (see p. 146). Alkanet is calming to the skin: insect bites are magically relieved if you pulp the fresh plant (stems, leaves, flowers, the lot), and pack onto skin. (It's also said to be good for eczema, as well as opening dirt-clogged pores and blackheads.)

If you can get hold of a plant or some seeds, put it in the sunniest, driest, sandiest spot in your garden (though it dislikes acid soils). It's a biennial, and so if you plant it, the deep, lapis lazuli blue flowers will appear from mid- to late summer the following year. (The leaves are hairy, a bit like borage; in fact, it's a member of the same plant family.) Alkanet can sometimes be found wild – it likes waste ground – so do keep your eyes peeled.

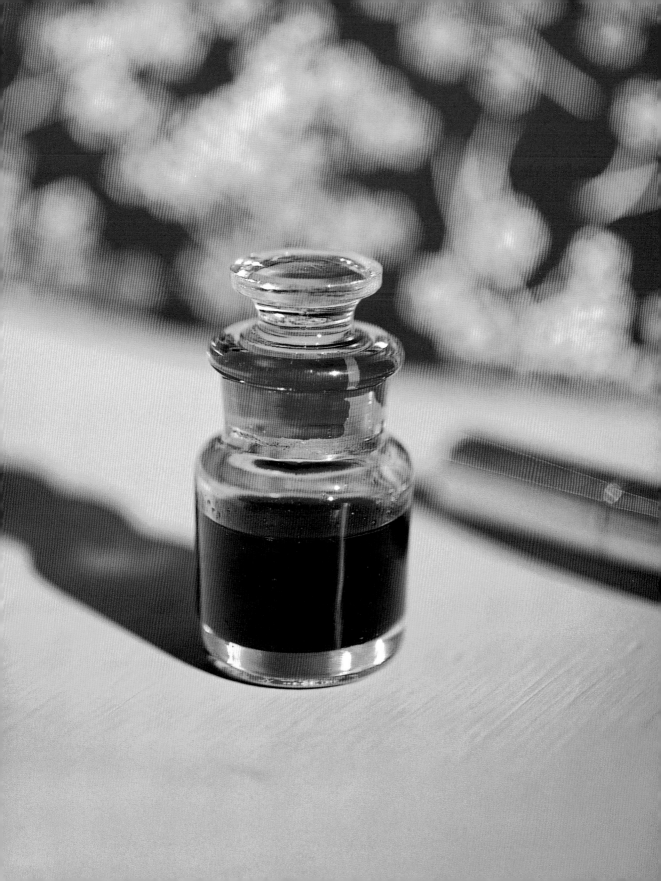

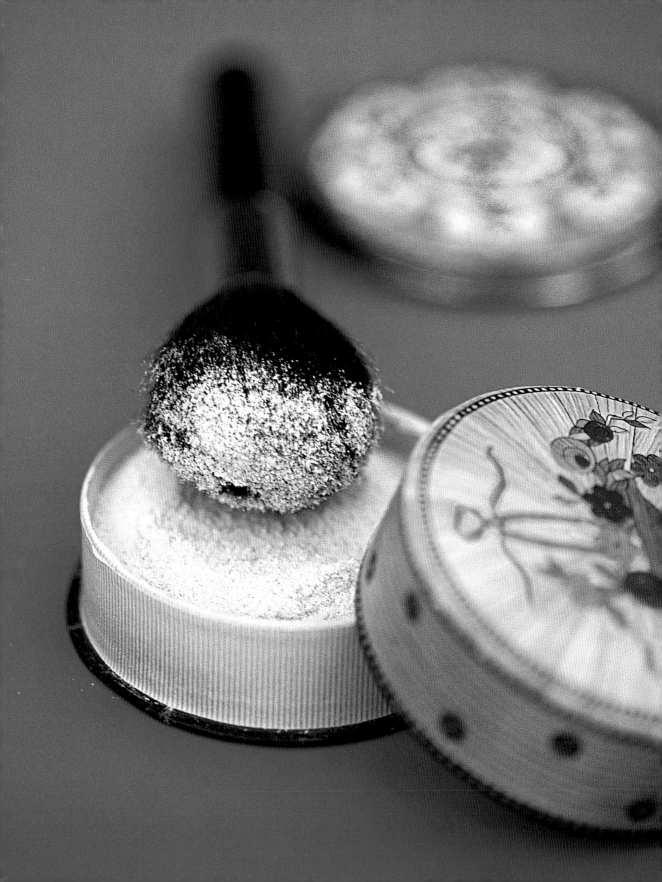

The low-down on talc

Most face powders contain talc, or magnesium silicate, which is a mined mineral. It has been associated with breathing problems, in some people – and now there are environmental concerns about it: in India, tiger habitats are (according to *Health WHICH?* magazine) being threatened by illegal talc mining. In addition, there are health question marks over the use of talc as a body powder – some health professionals believe that there may be possible links with ovarian cancer. Certainly, if you do choose to use any talc-based product, you should hold your breath while it's in the air – and don't ever use it to powder your female 'bits'!

fabulous face powder

Try using this scented face powder to 'fix' foundation or whenever your skin gets shiny.

10g (¹/₂oz) rice powder
25g (1oz) orris root powder
25g (1oz) dried lavender flowers

Put all the ingredients together in a screw-top jar and shake, shake, shake. Do this every day for 1–2 weeks, then put the powder in a sieve and sift into a bowl. Do not crush the lavender flowers; you want them simply to infuse the powder with their fragrance. Apply to skin with a velvet puff or a soft brush.

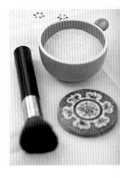

TIP

You don't always need powder to keep shine at bay. If your skin gets oily or starts to gleam, pull apart the two layers of a tissue, and lay one over the T-zone (which is where shine tends to develop). Gently press onto skin, and you'll find that the oil is lifted off, without the need to add another layer of powder.

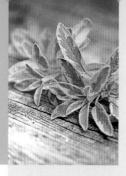

sage lash conditioner

This oil can also be stroked along brows to add lustre. The sage can also have a slightly darkening effect, so you may find you don't need so much mascara or brow pencil, after using for a while.

25g (1oz) fresh sage leaves or 10g (1/2oz) dried sage)
75ml (3fl oz) filtered, mineral or rainwater
2 tablespoons extra virgin olive oil

Put the sage and water in a pan, bring to the boil then simmer for 10 minutes. Cool and strain through a muslin cloth or kitchen paper. Put 1 tablespoon of the *tisane* into a small-necked bottle; add the olive oil and give the bottle a good shake. (You'll need to shake the bottle before use each time to mix the oil and water elements.) Apply the conditioning mixture each night to eyelashes using a clean mascara wand. (Wash and rinse the wand after use to ensure it's sterile; leave to dry on a radiator or near a towel rail).

TIP

Though I tried experimenting with creating a home-made mascara for this book, I just wasn't happy with the results. So my suggestion, if you want a natural-as-possible mascara, is to go for Dr Hauschka's, which smells wonderfully of roses, and is very comfortable to wear – though be aware it's not at all waterproof.

SAGE
Salvia officinalis

There are dozens of different sages. (You could plant an entire herb garden with sage alone.) For beauty-seekers, this wonderfully aromatic herb can be used for its ultra-soothing and astringent, oil-busting power in deodorants, face products, shampoos. As a hair rinse, it naturally darkens while delivering a glossy sheen – and it's a great dandruff-blitzer, too. Let running water rush into your bath through a muslin bag of sage, meanwhile, and it'll have a pick-you-up effect. Sage is a smile-brightener, too: as long ago as 1779, it was mentioned in *The Toilet of Flora* as an ingredient in a tooth-cleanser.

Grown in the garden, sage is unfussy, and just as happy in a pot as in the ground, but you'll need to replace the plant every few years if it gets leggy. Herbal lore says the best time to harvest sage is just before flowering – herbalists recommend doing this just before noon. (It has medicinal properties, too: sage tea, sweetened with honey, is good for sore throats and chestiness.) No beauty garden should be without it.

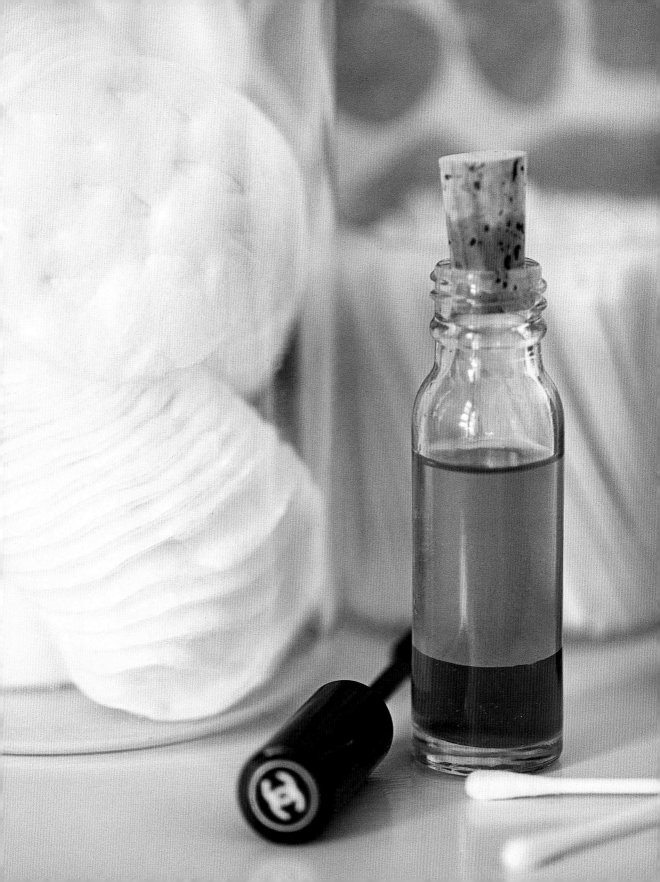

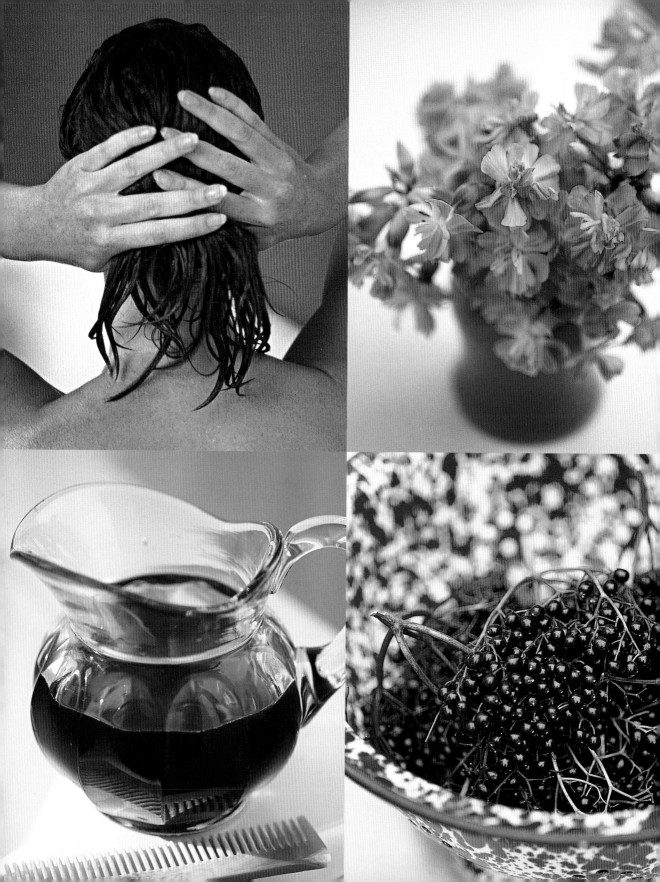

hair

Modern shampoos often contain harsh, oil-stripping detergents which can irritate the scalp and allow other synthetic ingredients to penetrate the body more easily. Some chemical hair dyes, meanwhile, also have a health question mark over them. (And the jury's still out about their long-term use.) But it's possible to **care for hair more gently** – with kinder shampoos, **shine-enriching treatments** and even colour-enhancing at-home treatments. **All 100 percent natural and botanically based**. So you'll know the **botanicals are in the bottle** – rather than simply a pretty picture on the label...

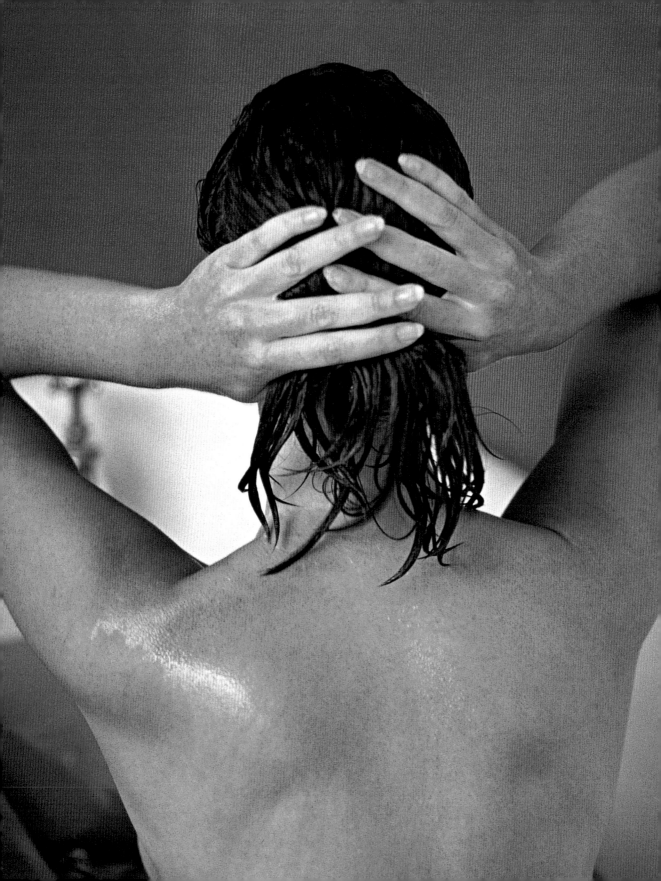

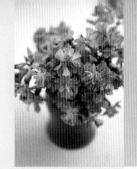

simple soapwort shampoo

SOAPWORT
Saponaria officinalis

The best advice I can give you about soapwort is: don't expect it to froth up exactly like your regular shampoo or body wash. But in reality – despite brainwashing from the world's shampoo barons – you don't need a mountain of foam to get skin, hair and scalp clean: soapwort does the trick perfectly well. Grown in the garden, soapwort has clusters of whiteish/pinkish flowers, which bloom throughout summer, and this perennial plant ultimately reaches 80 cm (30 inches) high. (Do watch out: soapwort, which grows wild in central and southern Europe on embankments and roadsides, can become a troublesome and surprisingly drought-resistant weed.)

Most often, it's the leaves or the rhizome-like roots that are used in cosmetics: they're gathered, washed clean and dried, either in sunlight or a very low oven (see p. 146), and then brewed into a decoction (see p. 153 for how to do that). You can buy dried soapwort if it's too much of a pain to grow, dry and harvest yourself – or alternatively, experiment with soap bark (*Guillaia saponaria*), from South America, which can be used in the same way. Be warned, meanwhile: if you get soapwort or soap bark in your eyes, it can irritate severely. (But then so do most shampoos.) Always rinse with your head tipped well back.

Use this in the same way as a normal shampoo. However, you'll need to use more of this than you would a detergent shampoo – and don't expect much of a lather; soapwort cleans without lots of froth. Keep the soapwort mixture out of your eyes as some people find it stings, and follow with a conditioner or herbal rinse.

2 tablespoons crushed fresh soapwort root or
*   1 tablespoon crushed dried soapwort root*
2 tablespoons of herbs (elderflower, fennel, horsetail, nettle
*   and rosemary are all herbs hair loves)*
5 drops of essential oil (lavender or – if you have a tendency to
*   dandruff – sage or rosemary)*
1.5 litres (2¹/₂ pints) filtered, mineral or rainwater

Pour the water over the soapwort root and the herbs in a pan and bring to the boil. Cover and simmer for 20–25 minutes. Remove from the heat and leave to cool thoroughly, then strain through a piece of muslin or kitchen paper over a sieve; press down to extract as much as possible of the herbs. Add the essential oils, drop by drop. Transfer to a sterilised glass bottle, shake and store in a cool, dry place out of sunlight.

Use around 200ml (7fl oz) each time you wash your hair; the technique is to wet your hair first, then pour the liquid into the palms of your hands and massage in well, until your hair is lathered lightly. Rinse thoroughly and repeat, if it's more than a few days since you've washed your hair. Follow with a final herbal rinse made as an infusion (see p. 153) from the same herbs that you used in the soapwort mixture. This quantity of soapwort shampoo keeps for just over 1 week, in the fridge – or you can freeze it in a plastic container and defrost as required.

quick oil solver

You know those times when you haven't the time to wash and style your hair, but it's sending out an S.O.S.? This sprinkle-on, shake-out treatment works like a dry shampoo, to absorb oil and make hair look and feel fresh again. It's best in a beauty emergency, rather than as a regular treatment, though.

25g (1 oz) powdered orris root
25g (1 oz) arrowroot powder
10 drops rosemary essential oil

Put the orris root and arrowroot in a screw-top sugar shaker and add the essential oil; shake to disperse the drops. Tip your head upside-down and brush your hair. Shake small amounts of the mixture onto the scalp and rub in (start at the base of the neck and work forward). Bend over at the waist and stroke and massage your scalp with the fingers; brush through with a bristle brush to absorb grease and leave hair smelling fresh. Do this over a towel, or outside, as it can get messy. (You can make your own orris root powder – but it takes a long time; orris is produced from the rhizomes of a beautiful garden plant, *Iris germanica florentina*, which are lifted, cleaned, left for three years and then pulverised to a powder, which smells deliciously of violets. If you can't wait that long – and I'm certainly much too 'I-want-it-now' for that – buy orris root powder instead, from a herbalist.)

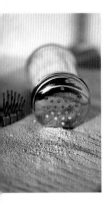

herb-boosted shampoo

Castile is the gentlest soap you can buy; it's basically a pure soap, which cleanses gently and efficiently and certainly isn't packed with chemicals that you may not care to expose your scalp to on a regular basis. Because soapwort shampoo is pretty time-consuming to make, I suggest turbo-charging the power of Castile soap with herbs, to help maintain hair health and very, very subtly enhance your natural hair colour (chamomile for fair hair, rosemary for dark hair, marigold for red hair).

10g (¹/₂oz) dried chamomile (for blondes), rosemary (for brunettes) or marigold (for redheads)
125ml (4fl oz) water
125ml (4fl oz) Castile shampoo
1 tablespoon vegetable glycerine
2 drops essential oil to match the herb of your choice

Make a strong infusion (see p. 153 for technique) of the herbs and the water. Then add to the shampoo and glycerine in a plastic jug or bottle (a clean, empty shampoo bottle is ideal); drop in the essential oils and leave to thicken overnight. Use like regular shampoo, and of course, rinse well after use.

TIP

If you want to stick to your usual commercial shampoo, you can still boost its herb power with this infusion.

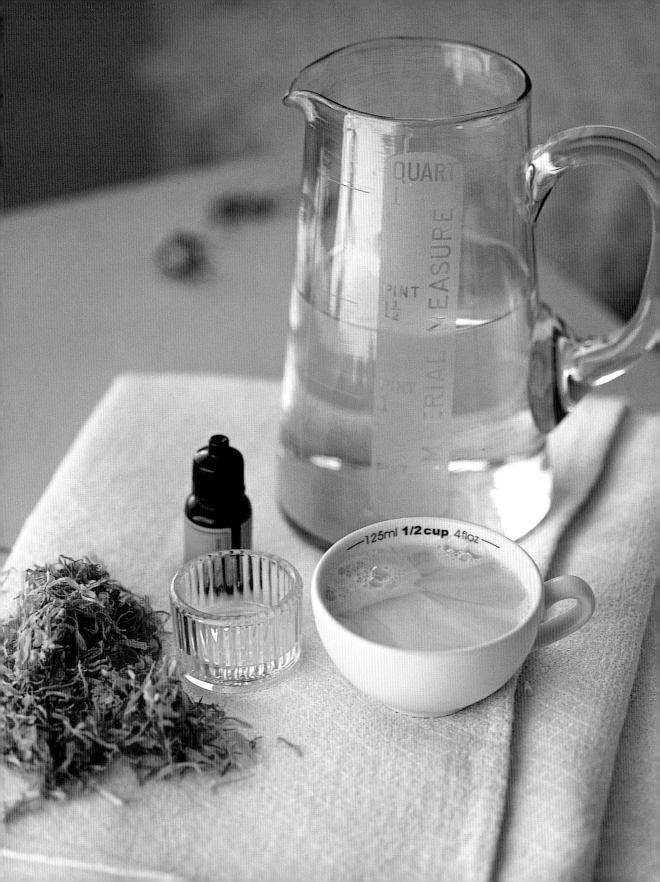

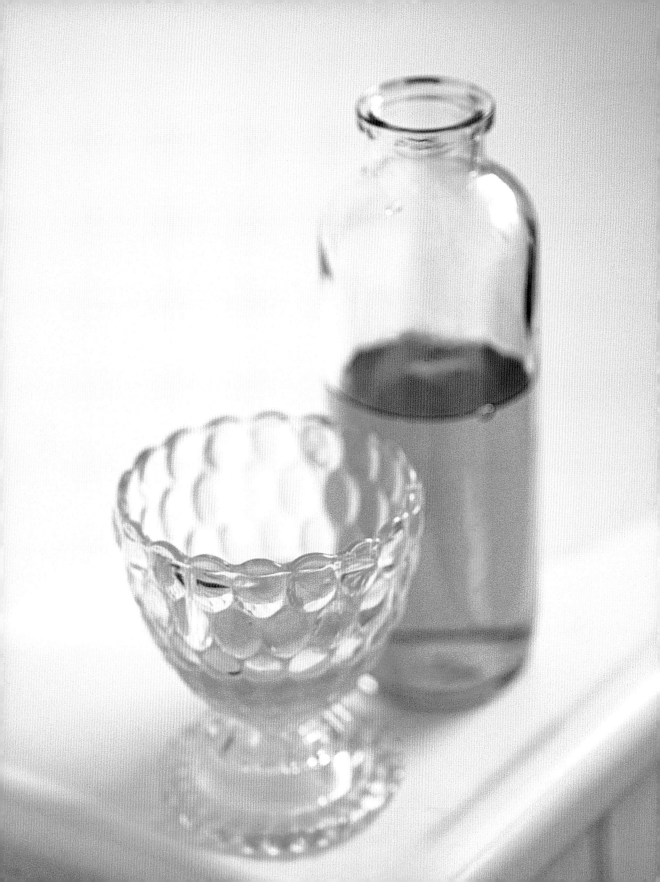

herbal hair shine treatment

If your hair has split ends, is brittle or otherwise out of condition, use a super-charged pre-shampooing treatment regularly to put back the gloss and shine. (Once a week is ideal.) If you have very long hair, this is sufficient for one treatment; if yours is short use less; it will keep well in the jar between treatments.

10g (¹/₂oz) rosemary leaves
10g (¹/₂oz) dried chamomile flowers
100 ml (3¹/₂oz) coconut oil

Chop the rosemary leaves and place in the top of a double-boiler (see p. 153) with the chamomile flowers and the oil and heat for 30 minutes; you may need to preheat the coconut oil, if it's solidified. Remove from heat, allow to cool and pour into a screw-top jar. Seal and leave for a week. Then heat again and strain through a sieve, to remove the herbs. To use the treatment, scoop the mixture out with your hands and work into scalp and hair; comb through from root to tip, if possible. Wrap your hair in a hot towel for 30 minutes. Then shampoo out the treatment (you'll probably need to shampoo twice) and condition hair; a capful of cider vinegar in the final rinse works as an effective conditioner.

nettle shine and volume rinse

The advantage of using fresh nettles is that they have a very long growing season. Wear thick gardening gloves for picking and chopping them!

50g (2oz) stinging nettles or 25g (1oz) dried nettles
125ml (4fl oz) cider vinegar
125ml (4fl oz) filtered, mineral or rainwater
6 drops rose essential oil

Finely chop the fresh nettles (if using). Put the nettles in the top of a double-boiler (see p. 153) with the vinegar and water. Cover and simmer for 1 hour (don't let the pan underneath boil dry). Cool, strain into a jug and add the essential oil drop by drop. Pour over washed hair, squeeze out the excess, then dry. Use as often as you like – it's amazingly shine-boosting.

cooling scalp saver

The only living part of the hair – the bulb – is rooted in the scalp, so it follows that for hair to look good, the scalp must be in optimum condition. This has all the right ingredients to cool, soothe and moisturise.

¹/₄ cucumber, peeled
150 ml (5fl oz) yogurt
1 heaped teaspoon honey

Liquidise the cucumber then mix with the yogurt and honey. Apply carefully to dry hair, smoothing it on so that every hair and your scalp are thoroughly coated. Leave for 10 minutes, then shampoo.

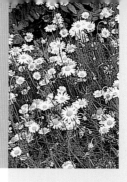

chamomile and rhubarb hair brightener

Used once a week, this will keep the summer lightness in blonde hair, or gradually lift mouse-to-fair hair.

25g (1oz) dried chamomile flowers
25g (1oz) powdered dried rhubarb root
200ml (7fl oz) boiling filtered mineral or rainwater
1 tablespoon extra virgin olive oil

In a pestle and mortar or an electric herb grinder, grind the chamomile flowers to a fine powder. Combine them with the powdered rhubarb root in a bowl. (See p. 146 for how to dry your own rhubarb root.) Add the boiling water to create a paste, and then mix in the olive oil. Using clips or grips, section off your dry hair and smooth the paste from roots to tip of each section. Wrap your hair in clingfilm and allow the treatment 45 minutes to work. Rinse thoroughly with warm water, then shampoo and condition.

TIP

Although lemon juice isn't great for hair condition, it's fantastic for creating highlights. Don't pour it all over: select some 'chunks' or big strands, and work a cotton wool pad dunked in lemon juice through to the tip. (Be careful not to get lemon juice on your scalp, though, as it can burn in the sun.) If you use a mirror, you can work on the same streaks throughout your holiday and really create a sun-kissed effect.

CHAMOMILE
Anthemis nobilis

Chamomile is one of the most useful herbs in the beauty world; its soothing, de-puffing and skin-strengthening benefits can be experienced in creams, lotions, hair products and bath oils. (It's the ultimate herb for wannabe-blondes to cultivate, because of its naturally hair-lightening effects.) The name comes from the Greek *kamai* (ground) and *melon* (apple) – because if you tread on chamomile, it wafts a wonderfully appley fragrance which is said to be beneficial to the nervous system. (We also call it 'Roman chamomile' – despite the Greek name – because the Romans are said to have introduced it to Britain; according to Culpeper, they used an oil from the flowers to anoint stiff joints, and poured a soothing infusion into their baths.)

If you have space, it's lovely to make a chamomile 'lawn': the mat-like growth quickly colonises, and in late summer, will be covered in blooms which are the plant's true beauty bounty.

Chamomile is generally used for its anti-inflammatory and anti-irritating effects, but just occasionally, some individuals prove allergic to chamomile – so, as always, do a 'patch test' before gaily slathering on your beauty creation. If you don't grow and harvest your own, the dried herb – which is also the most widely used plant material in herbal medicine – retains its effectiveness very well. The bonus? A wonderfully sedative tea of dried chamomile flowers can be brewed to waft you sleep-wards.

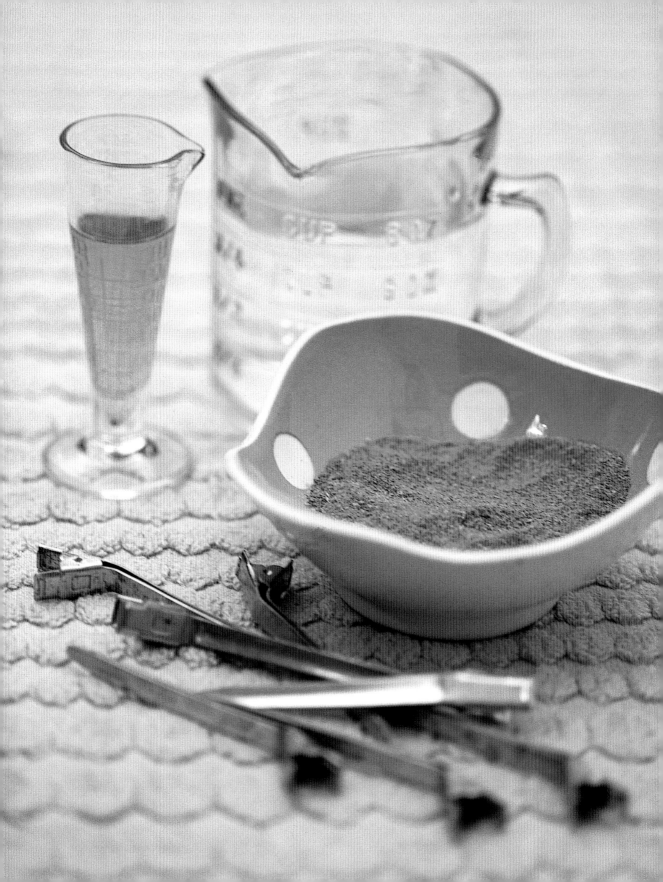

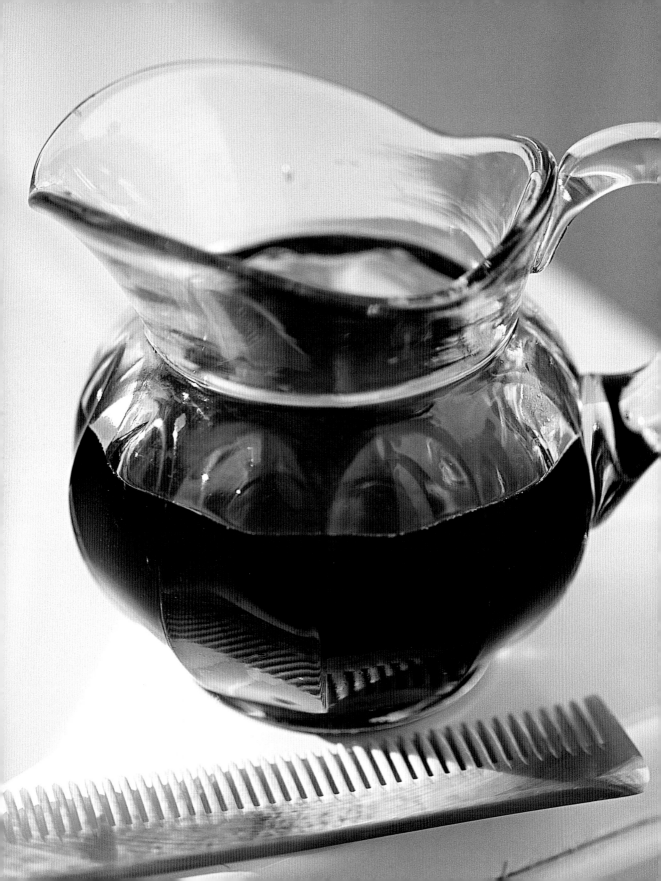

sage darkening treatment

Unfortunately, it's hard to find a botanical, 'back-garden' hair colourant that will cover grey hair – but this comes closest; it you use it regularly, it will gradually darken grey hair, though it won't ever cover it completely.

*110g (4 oz) chopped fresh sage leaves or
    50g (2 oz) dried sage leaves
225ml (8fl oz) cider vinegar
kaolin powder to mix
1 egg yolk (for a conditioning effect, if you like)*

Simmer the sage in the vinegar for 10 minutes and then strain while still warm. Allow to cool then sift in the kaolin, using a tea strainer or a sieve, until the mixture has a mask-like consistency. Gradually beat in the egg yolk. Using clips or grips, section off your dry hair and smooth the paste from roots to tip of each section. Wrap your hair in clingfilm and leave the treatment on for anywhere from 30 minutes to 1 hour. (A warm towel over the clingfilm can help speed up the treatment slightly.) Rinse with cool-to-warm (but not hot) water, and shampoo and condition. Use once a week.

If your hair tends to be dry and frizzy, you can also blend in 1 tablespoon olive oil to the mixture, after the egg yolk.

elderberry rinse for dark hair

Elderberries aren't in season all year round, of course, which is why I've given the Sage Darkening Treatment as an alternative. (Or why not freeze some?) You can also use leftover red or white wine for this recipe – if you don't always finish a bottle, keep a 'slop' bottle and pour the leftovers into it for use in your hair rinse.

*3 handfuls elderberries
600ml (1 pint) cider vinegar*

Put the elderberries and vinegar in a pan and bring to the boil. Simmer for 30 minutes. Remove from the heat; allow to cool before straining. Use as the final rinse, after washing your hair. This is enough for 1 treatment.

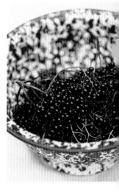

TIP

To make hair look lustrous, nourish it from within. Hair likes vitamin B complex (find it in brown rice and blackstrap molasses), as well as vitamin A (from orange and yellow vegetables and fruit, and dark green, leafy veg) plus iron (which, handily, is also found in blackstrap molasses, wholewheat and brown rice).

here come the reds

Used regularly, this will gradually and subtly add pretty red tones to your hair. (Beware if you bleach your hair, though, as this can make it go carrot-y.)

25g (1 oz) dried sage leaves
20g (³/₄oz) dried marigold leaves
225ml (8fl oz) red wine
kaolin powder to mix
1 tablespoon extra virgin olive oil
1 egg yolk

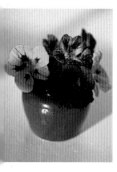

Put the sage and marigold leaves in a heatproof bowl and heat the wine in a small pan until just boiling. Pour it over the herbs then leave to cool thoroughly. Strain the herb-infused wine and then reheat in a clean pan. Using a tea strainer or a small sieve, slowly sift the kaolin powder into the wine, stirring constantly, until it has a mask-like consistency. Add the olive oil, which acts as a conditioner, and the egg. (Be sure the mixture is cooled before you do this, or it can scramble!)

Using clips or grips, section off your dry hair and smooth the paste from roots to tip of each section. Then wrap your hair in clingfilm and leave on for at least 45 minutes. (You can put a warm towel over the clingfilm, if you like.) Rinse out with plenty of warm water, then shampoo and condition.

Red hair also loves...

Ginger powder and juniper berries; you can also make a decoction from nasturtiums (see p. 93), and use this as a final rinse.

Hibiscus flowers also give red highlights to light or dark hair, and will enrich natural red. Make a tisane (see p. 153) from the flowers (or you can buy hibiscus teabags); allow to cool and strain before using as a final rinse.

Cranberry juice also works as a natural brightener for red hair, enhancing its brightness and smoothing the cuticles, so it looks shinier. Be sure to use unsweetened cranberry juice, though, or it will leave your hair sticky.

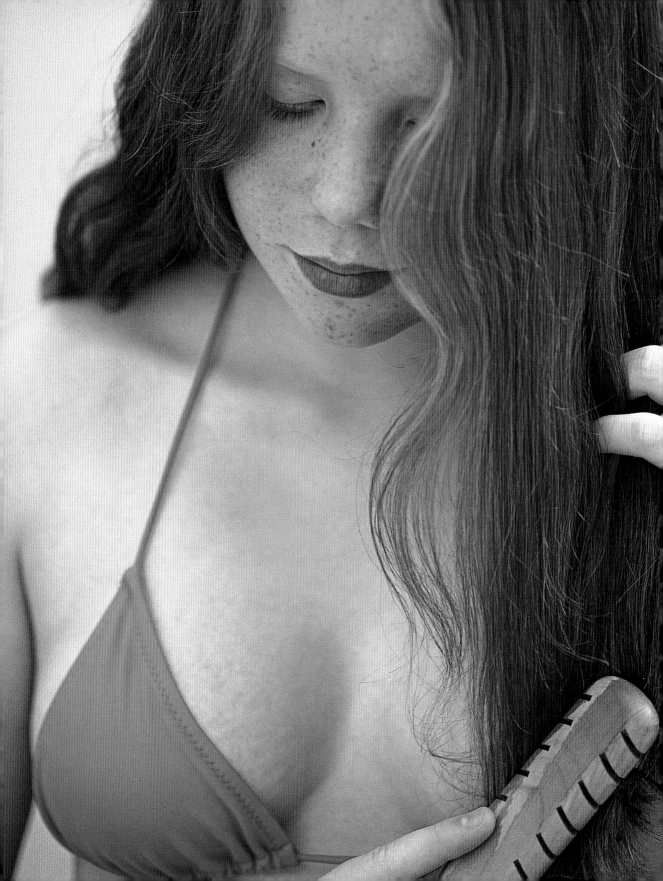

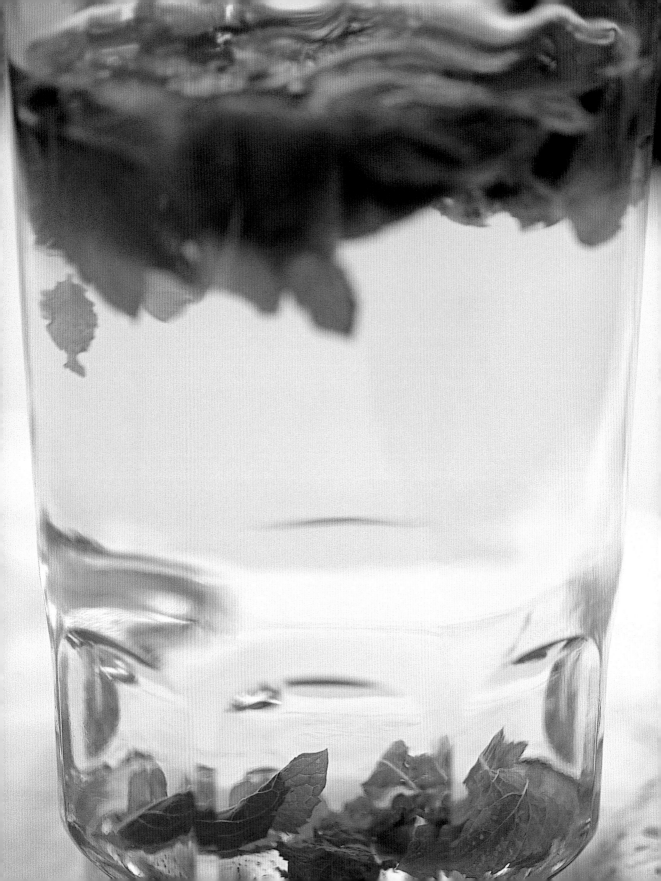

invigorating mint tea rinse

Why not drink a refreshing cupful, while you're at it? Very uplifting.

2 large handfuls fresh mint leaves
600ml (1 pint) boiling filtered or mineral water

Pour the boiling water over the mint and leave to stew. When the liquid has cooled, strain the mint and discard. Wash hair as normal and use the mint tea as a final conditioning rinse; comb while still wet and dry hair as usual.

TIP

Did you know that you can use raw egg in place of shampoo? Wet hair, massage a whole egg into your scalp and hair, and then rinse out with cool or warm water (but not hot, or you'll end up with a scrambled scalp...) Eggs are great natural shine-boosters for any hair type.

apple juice dandruff blitzer

Dandruff shampoos are harsh, medicinal – and are very stimulating to the scalp, whereas I believe it should be soothed and calmed. Apple has an antiseptic action and you can use this as a rinse to help rebalance the scalp and tackle your dandruff problem in a natural, healing way.

1 kg (2¹/₄ lb) fresh apples or
600ml (1 pint) bottled apple juice (sugar-free)
600ml (1 pint) filtered, mineral or rainwater
125ml (4fl oz) cider vinegar
5 drops tea tree essential oil
2 drops lavender essential oil

Juice the apples (or take the bottled juice) and mix with the water. Add the vinegar and essential oils, drop by drop, and swish. Once you've rinsed and/or conditioned the hair, use this as your final rinse. Contrary to expectation, it doesn't leave hair sticky!

TIP

Nasturtium is widely used by French herbalists for many scalp problems, from weakened hair to a scalp that's out of whack. To make a simple decoction (see p. 153) of the flowers, leaves and stems, take several really good handfuls, cover with water and boil for 10 minutes. Strain and use the liquid as a final rinse.

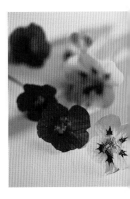

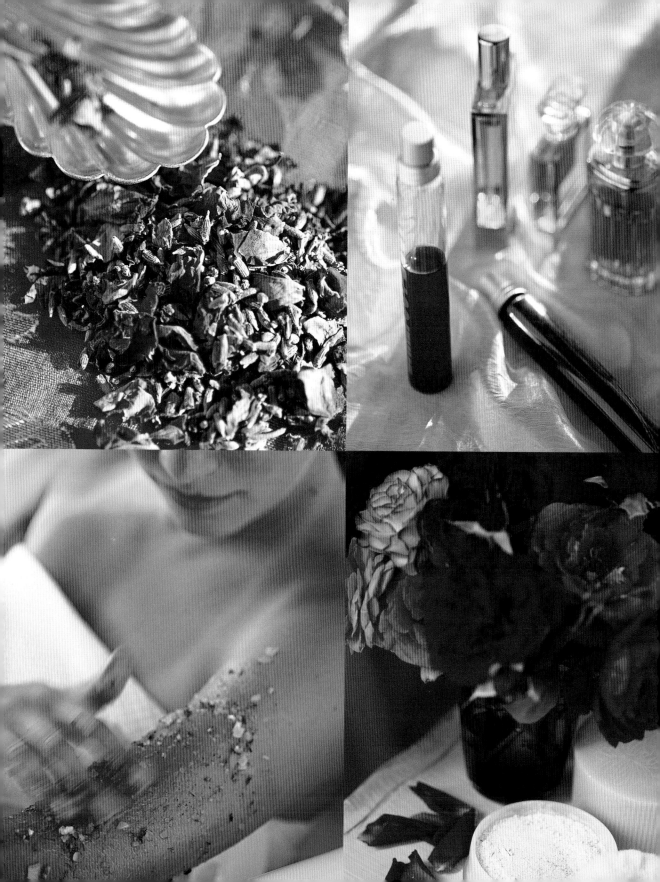

bath and body

The **skin on your body** soaks up a lot of what you put on it – and what you bathe in. Apply a moisturising body lotion – and **where does it go**? Some of it, for sure, goes into the bloodstream. Meanwhile, do you really want to wallow in a soup of synthetic chemicals, in the tub? I don't. But when it comes to nourishing parched body skin, or **mood-shifting bath additives**, or dusting on a sensual veil of powder, there are **botanical alternatives**. Heavenly to use. **Balm for the senses**. And – especially if you are able to buy or grow your own organic ingredients – as natural as it's possible for bathing and body treats to be…

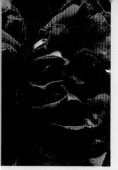

roses, roses, roses everywhere

This wonderfully luxurious bath is, quite simply, balm for the senses. I would never have believed it till I tried it myself and felt utterly transported from reality after a stressful day at the computer. (For fun, I put a dark red rose petal on each eyelid, which worked surprisingly well as an eye mask to dim the light level.) The one downside of this bath is cleaning it afterwards; swish with the shower head and the petals will collect in the plughole, where they can be scooped out. (Trust me: it's worth the extra housework.)

125ml (4fl oz) rosewater
1 tablespoon sweet almond oil
5 drops rose essential oil
75g (3oz) unsprayed rose petals (any kind, but scented roses
  are preferable)

Combine the rosewater with the sweet almond oil in a bottle and then add the rose essential oil, drop by drop. Pour this under running taps and throw the rose petals into the bathwater.

You can, of course, dry rose petals in summer to enjoy this bath year-round; the best roses to choose are Gallica roses (*Rosa gallica officinalis*), as these hold their fragrance even when dried.

ROSE
Rosa centifolia and
Rosa gallica

Every beauty garden should have swags of roses growing wherever there's space – because rose is a wonderfully versatile ingredient. Lately, it seems to have been rediscovered by the mainstream beauty industry, big-time, for its rejuvenating and restorative powers, which can benefit skin that's been damaged by scars, acne and sun. It is gentle on skin, too, making it ideal for sensitive skins. The petals can be scattered in the bath, or used to make an eye compress, or even to concoct a cheat's rosewater (see p. 18), while Culpeper said that an ointment of roses would cool and heal red pimples on the face. Personally, as well as growing masses of roses for their petals, I wouldn't want to be without rose and rose otto essential oil (organic for preference) for fragrancing the cosmetics I make at home.

Do try to use only home-grown, unsprayed roses in your home-made beauty treats; commercial roses are often as not drenched in pesticides. If you dry petals yourself, pick them in the early morning while the dew's still on them (just as they do in Grasse, home of the French perfume industry). Dry the petals on a large tray, out of direct sun, or you can put the tray in the airing cupboard to speed up the process. Store the dried petals in closed containers out of direct sunlight, to retain their bewitching scent and potency.

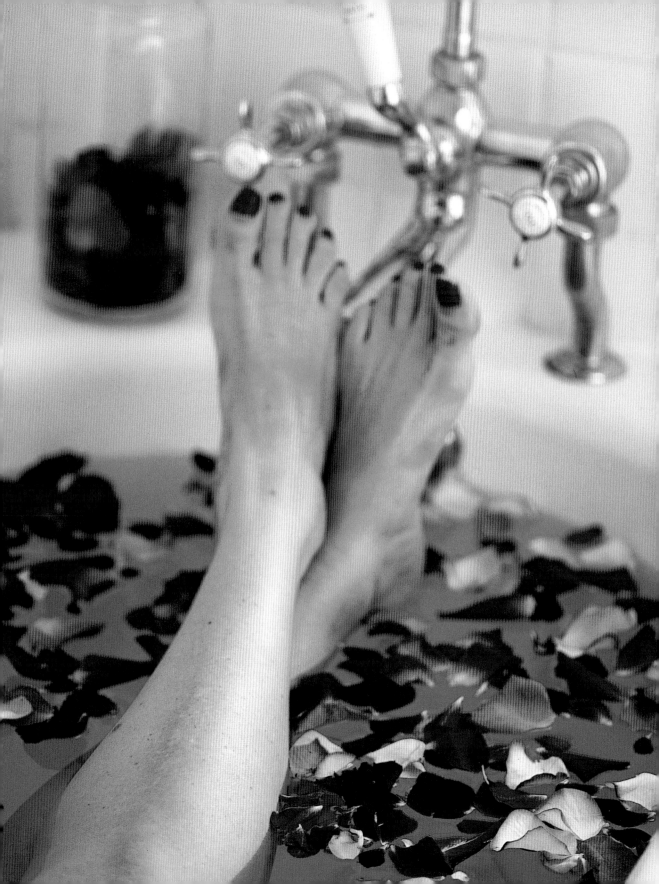

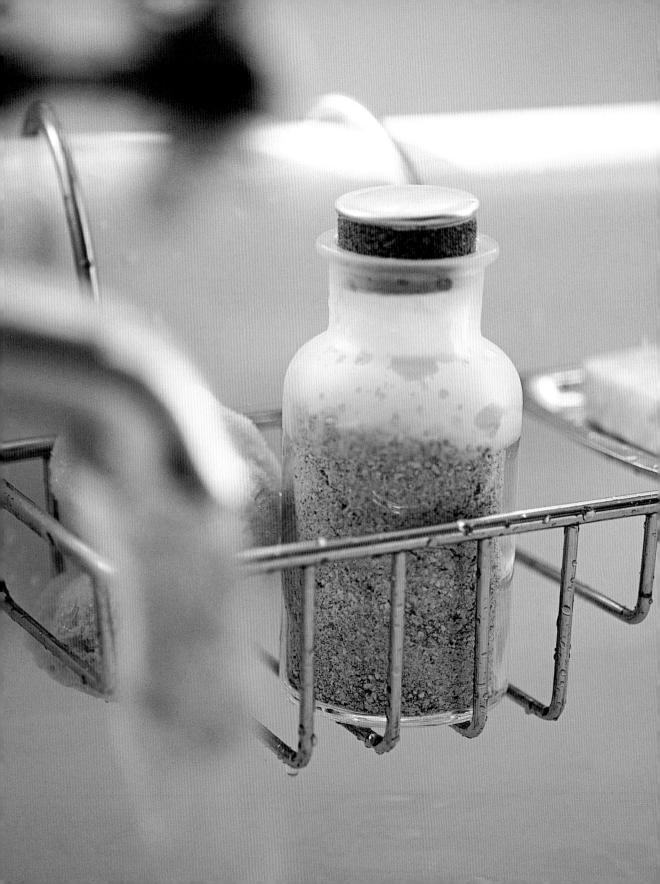

balancing lavender soak

The salt and bicarbonate have a water-softening effect, while the oatmeal is super-soothing for sensitive skins (and even for eczema).

100g (3¹/₂oz) dried lavender flowers
200g (7oz) oatmeal
50g (2oz) bicarbonate of soda
75g (3oz) salt

Put all the ingredients in a blender, and whizz until they become a fine-textured powder. The tiny lavender particles look very pretty in the jar, but if you like, you can add another small handful of the dried flowers at the end. Transfer into a storage jar that can be sealed with a cork, or has a screw-top, to keep the ingredients fresh. Pour around half a cupful under the running taps. To enhance the lavender fragrance, you can add up to 6 drops of essential lavender oil to each bathful and swish well.

TIP

Milk also makes an ideal additive for itchy, scratchy or dry skin; add 1–2 cupfuls – say up to 225ml (8fl oz) – fresh (or dried, reconstituted) milk to your bathwater. It is also great for dispersing essential oils; add 4–5 drops of your favourite oils per cupful before swooshing into the water.

elderberry bath tonic

Elderberry has a stimulating and tonic effect, and is soothing for inflammations, too. Pick the berries in late summer as they freeze successfully.

110g (4 oz) elderberry leaves and fruits
900ml (1¹/₂pints) filtered, mineral or rainwater
10 drops rose essential oil
4 drops rose geranium essential oil

Roughly chop the leaves and put in a pan with the berries and water and bring to the boil. Simmer for 5 minutes, then remove from the heat and allow to cool completely. Drop the essential oils into the bottom of a sterilised bottle and strain the liquid through a funnel lined with muslin or kitchen paper into the bottle. Add a cupful to the bath whenever you need a pick-me-up, and in between times, keep it in the fridge.

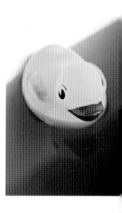

herbal bath bags

These bags can either be tossed in the tub – or, for best results, tied around the tap so that the rushing water pours through the herbs, to fill the bathroom with herbal steam: then soak the bag in the water, once you're in it. The bags can be untied and the contents left in the sun to dry, retied and used once or twice.

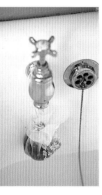

25cm (10 inch) square muslin or
*   cheesecloth for each bag*
ribbon, string or raffia
up to 50g (2oz) dried herbs or
*   other ingredients of your choice*
2–3 drops essential oil (to match
*   the herbs)*

Cut out a circle about 25cm (10 inches) radius from your cloth. Crush the herbs slightly to release their potency, heap them in the centre of the cloth and tie with a 45cm (18 inch) length of ribbon. On the second and third use, add 2–3 drops of essential oil to the dried herbs, to enhance the scent (rosemary if you use rosemary, sage if you use sage, and so on). Experiment with different 'bulk' ingredients alongside the herbs; use a total of about 50g (2 oz) of herbs and/or other ingredients per bag. Oatmeal is a very gentle ingredient, but it's not the only skin-friendly possibility. Ground almonds or dried milk powder can also be added, or for a powdery sweet fragrance, use dried orris root. You can even use polenta! Also, try rubbing the muslin or cheesecloth over your skin to lightly exfoliate and apply the herbal ingredients topically and maximise their benefits.

herbal bath teas

As an alternative to bath bags, you can brew a herb infusion and (when cooled), pour this into the bath. (See p. 153, but use around 2 cups dried herbs to 600ml (1 pint) boiling water).

For fragrance, use sweet-scented herbs like rose, lavender, meadowsweet, violet, jasmine, carnation, honeysuckle or rose geranium. Combine these with spicy herbs (chamomile, eau-de-cologne mint, clary sage, lovage, rosemary and lemon balm). For soft skin, use cleansing, soothing ones – chickweed, sage, cowslip, marshmallow, marigold, pansy, apple mint, spearmint, elderflower, red clover, comfrey or fennel seed. I like to create what I call my 'magic bath' – a bit of this, a bit of that – depending on my mood and what's fresh in the garden.

Here are some other effective bath bag recipes – but have fun experimenting. **Rose petals** and **lavender** are good for a sensual soak. **Rosemary, bay, basil, thyme, sage** and **lemon verbena** invigorate a tired body and weary mind. **Peppermint** and **lovage** are naturally deodorising and blissfully cooling in hot weather. **Lime flowers, chamomile, lemon balm** and **valerian** soothe and relax at bedtime. **Grated ginger** works wonderfully to ease aches and pains. **Strawberry leaf, burdock** and **chamomile** also make a good combination. **Peppermint, thyme, dandelion** and **sage** are excellent for purifying blemished or oily skin on the body. **Myrtle** is good for cellulite and/or for toning slack skin.

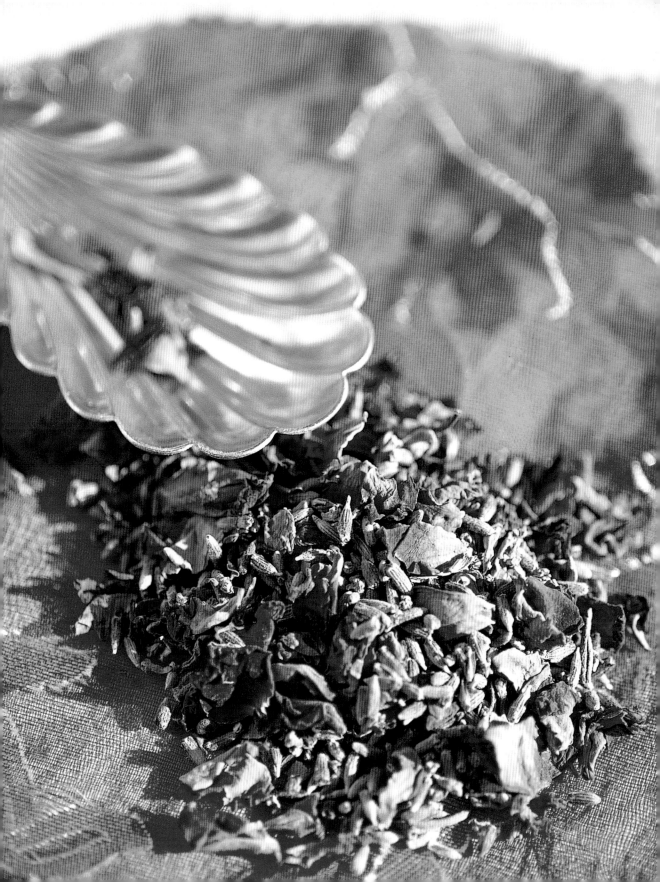

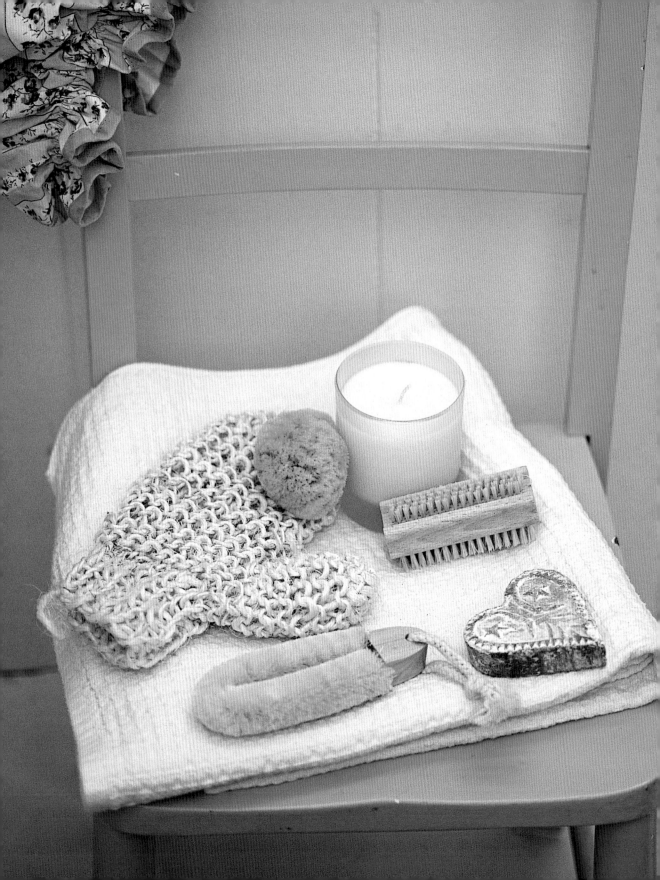

at-home spa essentials

If you want to turn your bathroom into paradise, stock up on the following:

- Large sea sponge (look for sustainably harvested on the label)

- Loofah

- Pumice stone

- Bath pillow

- Aromatherapy candle

- Large cotton towels

- Pretty bath cap

- Body brush/sisal washcloth

- Natural olive oil-based soap

TIP

To ease muscle aches, try an Epsom salts bath. Epsom salts – magnesium sulphate – are a natural muscle and nervous system relaxant, easing sore joints and muscles. Just throw 2 handfuls of Epsom salts into a hot bath, and soak yourself for 15 minutes.

purifying mud pack

No getting away from it: this is messy. Marvellously messy. In an ideal world, you'd drag an easy chair into the corner of the bathroom and line it with old towels; relax into the chair and let the mud work its magic. Otherwise you can put thick plastic over everything that might get mud-splashed – but it's much less sensual and enjoyable. The mud washes out of the towels easily on a hot wash with a good washing powder. (Nevertheless, I still wouldn't use my best towels for this…)

25g (1oz) fresh or dried lavender flowers
25g (1oz) fresh marigold (calendula) flowers (or 4 teaspoons dried)
25g (1oz) fresh scented rose petals (or 4 teaspoons dried)
225ml (8fl oz) very hot water
2 teaspoons yogurt
1 tablespoon honey
20g (³/₄oz) kaolin clay
1 teaspoon powdered liquorice root
5 drops neroli essential oil
5 drops rose essential oil
125ml (4fl oz) seawater (or mineral water with 2 teaspoons sea salt)
60g (2¹/₂oz) sea salt

Put the petals in a jug, and steep for at least 30 minutes in the hot water. Strain through muslin, kitchen paper or a fine sieve; set aside. Make a smooth paste with the yogurt and honey. Slowly add the kaolin, the liquorice root and the essential oils, and whisk so that the mixture doesn't go lumpy. Run a very hot bath (to steam up the room) and add the herb-infused water and the sea salt. Add the seawater (or your home-made version) to the original paste, and whisk again. Massage the mud mix onto your skin – this can be slathered on top-to-toe, though avoid your eyes and mouth area. After 10 minutes, sink into the bath and lie in the muddy water for 10 more minutes. (Test first to see if you need to add any more cold water.) Rinse yourself – and the bath – with cool water.

lavender and salt body scrub

Salt is a super-effective exfoliator and leaves skin invigorated. Sugar (see below) is gentler and it doesn't sting if you've scratched yourself!

150g (5oz) salt (I prefer Maldon salt but you can use any grainy salt: crystal or sea salt, kosher salt or Dead Sea salt)
100g (3¹/₂oz) dried or fresh lavender flowers
375ml (12fl oz) sweet almond oil
25 drops lavender essential oil

Blend the dry ingredients and place in a sealable jar (one with a rubber seal is ideal). Pour the oil over them. Depending on the type of salt you use, you may need to add a little more oil to top up the jar. Use by the handful, applied in circular strokes everywhere except the face, which is way too fragile. Rinse or shower off.

sugar-sweet body scrub

150g (5oz) sugar (I like golden granulated but white is fine)
25g (1oz) dried fennel seeds
375ml (12fl oz) sweet almond oil
20 drops sweet orange essential oil
5 drops ylang-ylang essential oil
5 drops patchouli essential oil

Mix the sugar and the fennel seeds in a bowl. Then tip into a large, sealable jar. Put the sweet almond oil in a jug, add the essential oils, and pour over the sugar. (You can vary the fragrance with your favourite essential oils, adding up to 50 drops of essential oil in total; this particular blend is pretty warm and sexy.) Add more sweet almond oil to top up the jar if necessary – this depends partly on the size of sugar granules. Use scoopfuls, in the bath, and massage into skin in a circular motion. Delicious… Rinse or shower off.

exfoliating loofahs

I always thought loofahs came from the sea – but in fact, these fibrous bath sponges can be grown in the garden, anywhere the growing season extends from early spring to late autumn. After the last frost, plant the flat gourd seeds in level ground, near a trellis the shoots can scramble up. The fruits will be ready to pick off the vine just before the first frost; then it's time to put them somewhere warm and dry until the outer skin becomes papery. Peel off the skin – and the sponge will be revealed. (Shake out the seeds, which can be planted next season.) Clean your new loofahs by soaking in 1 part bleach to 3 parts water, and then rinse them in clean, warm water until the last of the bleach has gone. Air-dry before use.

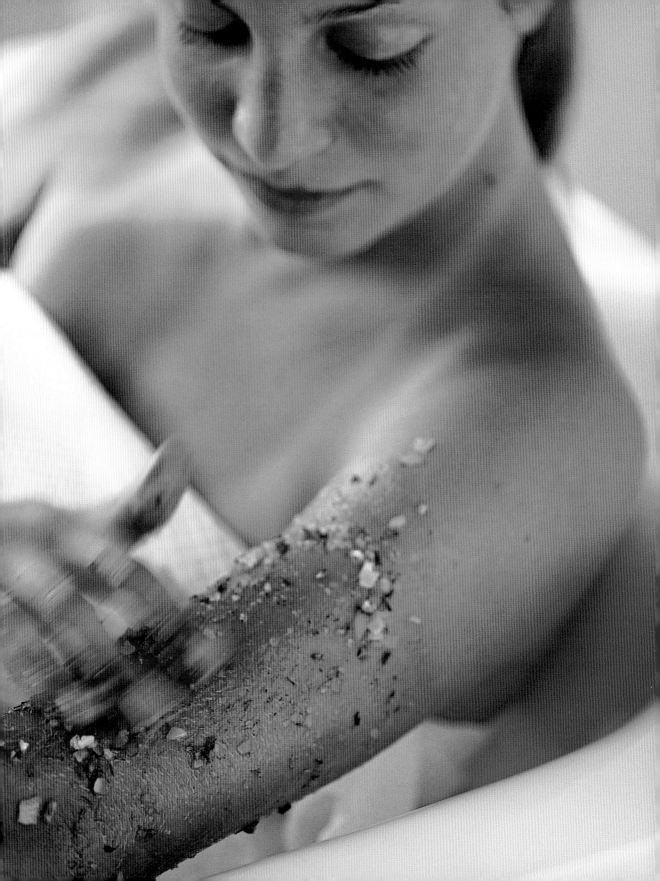

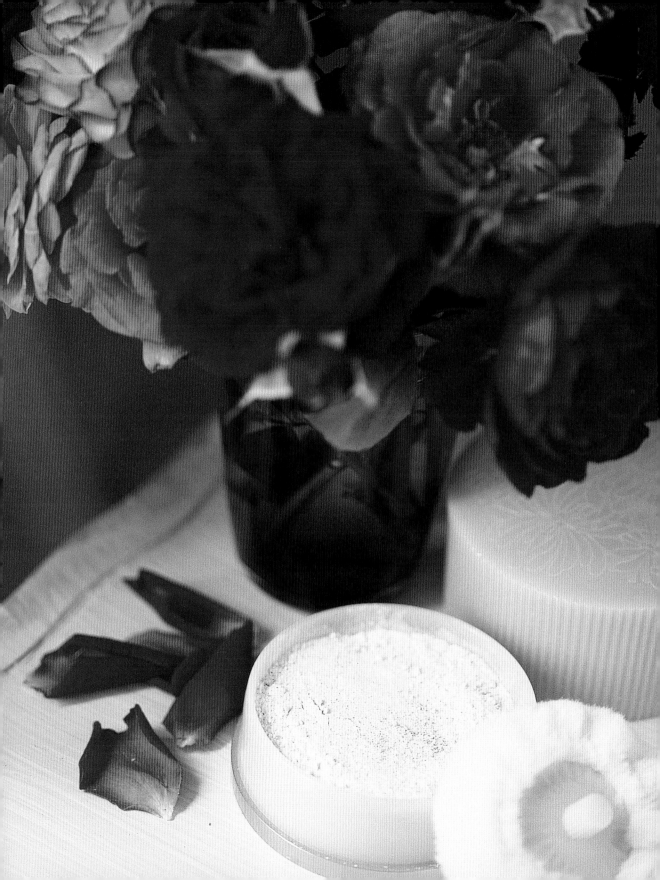

rose petal and lavender dusting powder

Personally, I prefer not to use talcum-based products; talcum is another product with a health question mark over it, if inhaled, as it's related to aluminium. Happily, I've found that botanical alternatives are just as effective. The roses and lavender become tiny coloured flecks in the powder.

110g (4oz) cornflour
55g (2oz) bicarbonate of soda
Approx 25g (1oz) dried lavender flowers
Approx 25g (1oz) dried rose petals
2 drops lavender essential oil
2 drops rose essential oil

Put all the dry ingredients in a food processor and whizz until you have a fine powder. Add the essential oil, drop by drop, and blend again; these enhance the fragrance. Then, using a sieve, shake the powder as if you were sifting flour, until it becomes a fine, soft texture. Put in a clean container and dust over your body using a powder puff – or put in a sugar shaker, and 'sift' onto your skin after the bath.

rose geranium body powder

My favourite variety of scented geranium would be 'Attar of Roses'. Dust this gorgeous powder onto your skin with a velvet puff or the kind of pretty, old-fashioned powder puff your granny used.

75g (3oz) cornflour
12 fresh scented geranium leaves, washed and dried
1 drop rose essential oil
2 drops rose geranium essential oil

Put the cornflour in a large screw-top jar, and add the essential oils and the geranium leaves. Screw on the lid tightly and shake to mix. Shake daily for 1 week, then remove the geranium leaves. Put the powder into a sugar shaker, for dusting, or a clean, dry box; use in place of talcum powder.

TIP

In summer, dust either of these body powders into your shoes to prevent them rubbing and giving you blisters.

love-in-a-mist body balm

Reputedly, the women of ancient Rome massaged their breasts at night with a tea or a powder made from nigella seeds – so if your *décolletage* is in need of some TLC, don't skimp.

50ml (2fl oz) rosewater
1/8 teaspoon borax powder
10g (1/2oz) love-in-a-mist (nigella) seeds, crushed
1 tablespoon grated beeswax
50ml (2fl oz) sweet almond oil
50ml (2fl oz) grapeseed oil
1 drop grapefruit seed extract
1 vitamin E capsule

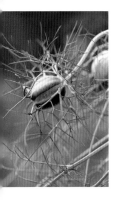

Heat the rosewater in a pan and add the borax. When the liquid just starts to boil, pour it over the love-in-a-mist seeds and allow to stand for 30 minutes to 1 hour, until cool. Heat the beeswax in the oils in the top of a double-boiler until melted (see p. 153). Strain the rosewater/borax liquid and reheat until it's around the same temperature as the oil/wax blend. (Use a thermometer for this, to take away the guesswork.) Pour the melted wax/oil mixture into a bowl, and very slowly add the rosewater/borax. Use a hand-held blender to mix until it becomes a smooth, thick lotion. Pierce the vitamin E capsule and add the oil. Pour into a screw-top jar. Use to massage well into dry patches of skin.

lady's mantle boob tonic

The firming action isn't just down to the coldness of the liquid – wise women used to prescribe lady's mantle (*Alchemilla mollis*) for breasts that were sagging from child-bearing or just plain old gravity's effects; a few weeks of this should make anyone's breasts Wonderbra-worthy again.

225g (8oz) lady's mantle leaves and/or flowers
600ml (1 pint) freshly boiled filtered, mineral or
    rainwater

Place the leaves and flowers in a large, heatproof bowl and pour over the boiling water to make a *tisane*. Steep for 10 minutes and allow to cool. Soak 2 muslin cloths – or face flannels – in the liquid, wring the excess back into the bowl and place the cloths over both breasts. Relax for 10–15 minutes. Pour the rest of the liquid into a screw-top jar and store in the fridge. Repeat daily.

TIP

Forget all that advice about applying body lotion or oil to damp skin to 'trap the moisture'. In fact, all you do is dilute what you're applying so it's less effective. Always pat your skin dry before applying creams and lotions.

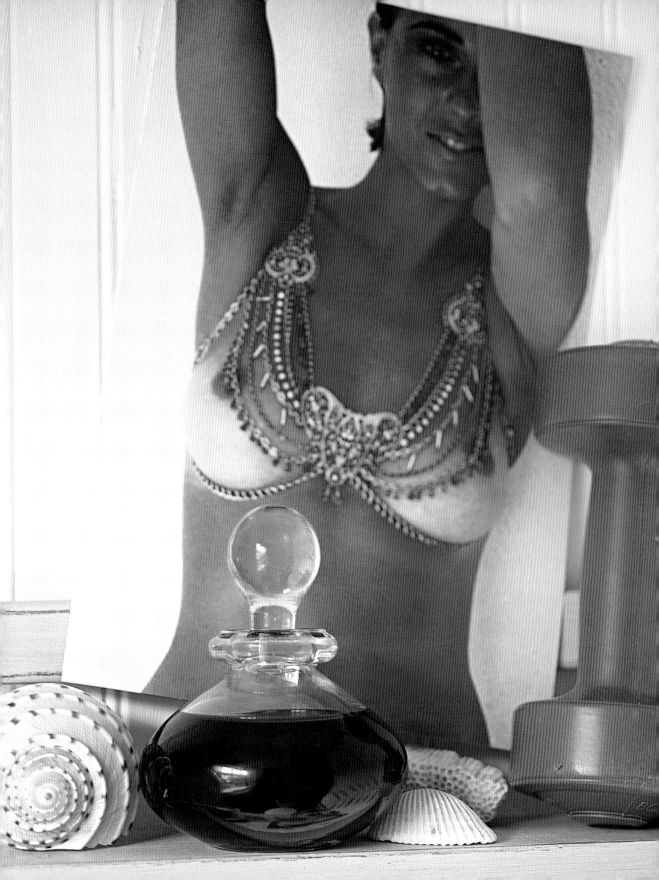

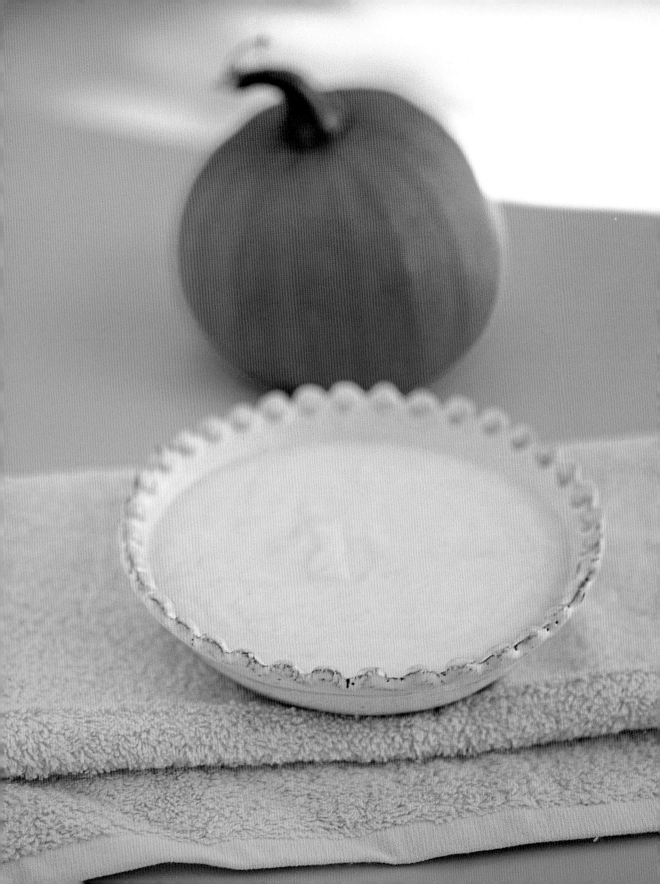

pumpkin body quencher

Pumpkin is a natural source of both fruit acids and vitamin A, which have a skin-brightening effect. In addition to making skin glow silkily, pumpkin allows other ingredients to soak in better.

1 small pumpkin
1 tablespoon sweet almond oil
Water
225ml (8fl oz) yogurt
1 lemon, juiced

Peel the pumpkin and cut off the top. Slice into quarters and scoop out the seeds and fibrous part from the middle (you can compost this). Cut the flesh into chunks. Put the pumpkin in a pan with a small amount of water and bring to the boil (keep an eye on it to ensure that it doesn't catch or boil dry). When it's soft, remove from the heat and mash with a potato masher. While still warm (but not hot), add the almond oil, the yogurt and the lemon juice.

In a warm bathroom, sit in the bath or stand in the shower – don't run the water yet – and slather yourself with the mixture. (Hair, too, if you like.) Sit for 10 minutes and then rinse or shower with warm water. Pat skin dry and apply moisturiser or body oil; shampoo and condition hair (if you used the 'quencher' on your hair, too).

cucumber body lotion

This is super-refreshing in hot weather. It's light rather than nourishing, so on areas of dry skin you might want to use a body butter instead. It also works well as a sinks-in-fast hand lotion, so keep it near the taps, and massage into hands after washing and drying them.

5 cm (2 inch) piece of cucumber, peeled
1 tablespoon witch hazel extract
1 teaspoon vegetable glycerine
1 teaspoon rosewater
2 drops grapefruit seed extract
5 drops rose or lavender essential oil (optional)

Chop and mash the cucumber in a pestle and mortar and add the witch hazel, glycerine and rosewater. (Alternatively, whizz the whole lot in a blender or food processor for 1 minute). At the last moment drop in the grapefruit seed extract and essential oil, if using, and whizz again. The result: a beautifully light, pale green lotion that rubs in easily. It should keep for a couple of weeks; make fresh after that.

TIP

Because cucumber juice gives a boost to all skin types, never discard the peel without rubbing it over your skin, inner side down – it's great for necks, arms, the back of hands, if you don't want to disturb your make-up.

111

body butter bliss

This is less messy to use than a liquid oil, as the beeswax transforms the oils into a solid butter. Use the 'maceration' technique on this page for the calendula oil (or use Neal's Yard Remedies' ready-made version).

1 tablespoon calendula-infused extra virgin olive oil
1 tablespoon coconut oil
2 tablespoons sesame oil
50g (2oz) grated cocoa butter
10g (1/2oz) beeswax
up to 20 drops of your favourite essential oils, optional

Put all the ingredients in the top of a double-boiler (see p.153) and heat gently until the beeswax has melted. Stir well, allow to cool slightly and pour the mixture into a sterilised jar with a screw-top. If you like, add a blend of your favourite essential oils once you've removed the mixture from the heat, and stir.

ultra-rich body oils

One of the best ways to harness the power of herbs is to macerate them in oil. Dr Mariano Spiezia, founder of one of my favourite beauty companies, Spiezia Organics (see RESOURCES, pp. 154–7), puts jars of herbal oils in sunlight (and moonlight!) for 2–3 weeks, before using the oils. Among the many herbs that can be used for maceration are: chamomile, comfrey, dandelion, fennel seed, scented geranium, lavender, lemon balm, marigold, marjoram, peppermint, rosemary, sage, thyme and yarrow. Dried herbs are best. For each oil, put 4 tablespoons herbs/flowers in a clear glass jar with a cork or screw-top. Cover with sweet almond, grapeseed or extra virgin olive oil. Ensure the herbs are completely submerged. Seal the jar and leave in a warm, sunny place for 10–15 days, and shake daily. (This increases the rate at which the active botanicals disperse into the oil.) Filter the oil, pressing it through muslin to extract the last drops of goodness from the herbs. Refilter, if required.

You are now ready to concoct your massage oil. For a relaxing blend, I suggest

4 tablespoons each of chamomile macerated oil,
marigold macerated oil, lavender macerated oil
and geranium macerated oil
5 drops chamomile essential oil (optional)
5 drops lavender essential oil (optional)

Pour the macerated oils into a bottle to blend, then add the essential oils (if using), drop by drop; shake very well and then allow the oil to settle again. This can be massaged into the body and is exquisitely, subtly aromatic, soothing and skin-replenishing.

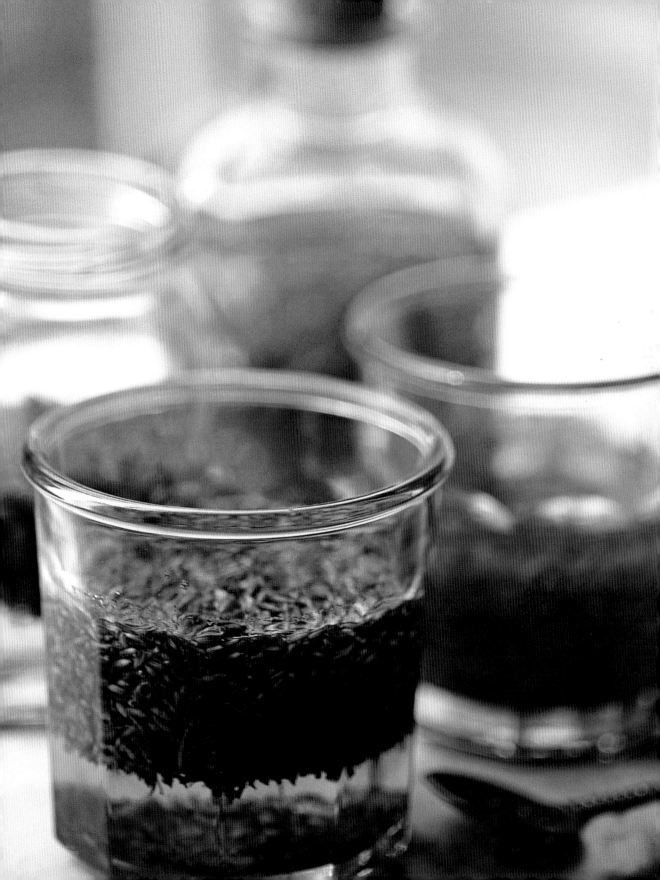

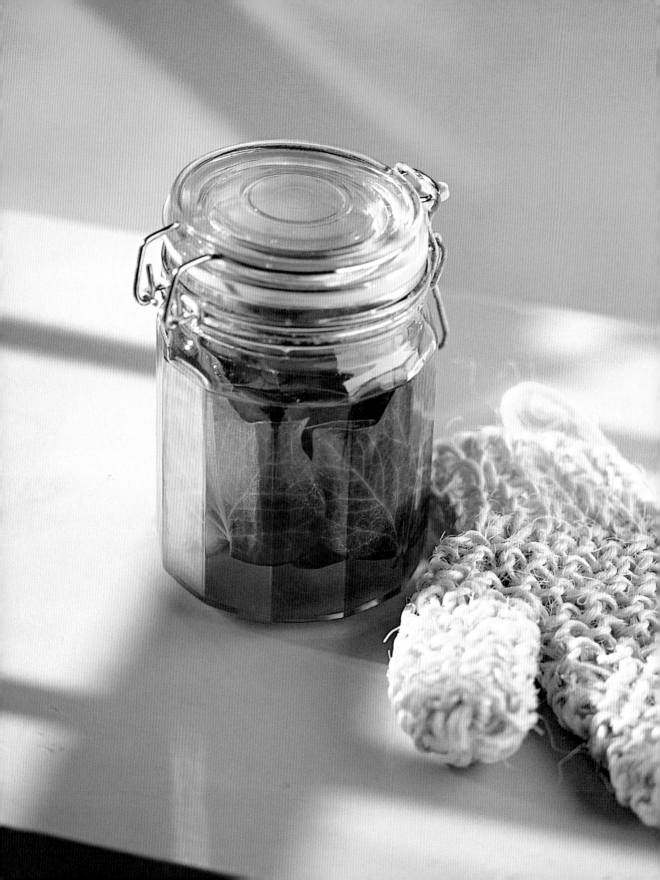

how to body brush...

After a couple of minutes of body brushing, you'll feel the same sense of exhilaration you get from a 20-minute walk. I swear by its power to slough away dead skin cells and boost circulation, and nobody I know who body-brushes regularly has a dimple of cellulite on their bottom, probably because it encourages elimination of toxins through the lymphatic system, helping to break down fatty pockets. Use a loofah, sisal mitt or a long-handled brush – be sure it's firm but not scratchy – and make long, upward, sweeping movements, starting at your feet and working up your legs and across your hips, bottom and tummy. Then move to your arms: beginning at your hands, move up your arms towards your shoulders, always working towards your heart. Resist the temptation to pummel thighs hard, or you can break tiny blood vessels – and if you have sensitive skin, wet the mitt and use it in the bath or shower with a natural soap or soapfree cleanser; the water reduces friction, minimising any damage. Try to get in the habit of body brushing every day: doing it regularly – rather than in occasional bursts – is what makes the difference.

ivy leaf anti-cellulite oil

Most of us can readily source ivy leaves, but if you should have a plant of butcher's broom (*Ruscus aculeatus*) growing in your garden, pick several sprigs of this and crush with the ivy leaves, before macerating in the oil. Butcher's broom, like ivy, is detoxifying, and can help shift cellulite.

15 large fresh ivy leaves
125ml (4fl oz) grapeseed oil
1 teaspoon wheatgerm oil
15 drops juniper essential oil
5 drops fennel essential oil
5 drops rosemary essential oil

Bruise the ivy leaves in a pestle and mortar, place in the bottom of a jar and pour the grapeseed oil over them. Add the other oils – the essential oils drop by drop. Leave the mixture for 1 week and then strain out the ivy leaves. Massage into problem areas – usually hips, thighs, bottom. Ideally, body-brush first, to maximise circulation. It looks pretty to line your storage jar with a few more ivy leaves, for decoration.

lavender deodorant

I've long had a hunch that there might be a link between breast cancer and the use of antiperspirants – sweat glands are, after all, the body's way of ridding itself of toxins and what happens if you trap them in the armpit…? So I actually gave up using antiperspirants ages ago. (Although I'm lucky: I never sweated much.) Now science is suggesting that there might, indeed, be a link between antiperspirants and breast cancer, and many women I know are giving them up. This deodorant is an effective alternative – and it doesn't block pores, so won't interfere with the body's natural detoxing process.

250ml (9fl oz) vodka
50g (2oz) dried lavender flowers
50g (2oz) fresh rose petals
10 drops lavender essential oil
10 drops rose essential oil

Pour the vodka over the flowers and petals and add the essential oils, drop by drop. Allow to infuse for 3 weeks, then strain and use in an atomiser in place of your regular deodorant. (Be warned: don't use on freshly shaved or depilated skin, as this will sting like crazy.)

TIP

If you're worried about B.O., and your problem persists even while using this deodorant, the cause may be clogged pores. When your body can't eliminate body wastes, bad body odour can result. So gently dry-brushing skin before every shower exfoliates the dead skin that traps odour-causing wastes. (For how to body brush, see the previous page.) This will improve circulation, which – in turn – will help your body detoxify more efficiently. (It might not fully eliminate your need for deodorant – but you should be able to use less of it.)

more natural pong-beaters…

Citrus peel gives skin a fresh, clean fragrance – but the citric acid in the peel also helps tackle bacteria on the skin's surface. Finely pare the outer peel from an orange or lemon (or half of each) in place of the lavender in the recipe here, and to enhance the fragrance, add 5 drops of sweet orange and 5 drops of lemon essential oil.

Lovage can be used in place of the lavender in the recipe on the left; this herb – which smells of celery – effectively cleanses and deodorises. (Use the fresh-picked herb.)

Rosewater is astringent and soothing; spritz it top-to-toe as a freshening mist (though it's less effective for serious B.O. than the other ingredients here).

Witch hazel is very effective for tightening underarm pores and deodorising too; on its own, it can be drying, so add 1 tablespoon vegetable glycerine to 50ml (2fl oz) witch hazel, and then add 10 drops of your favourite essential oils: rose, lavender, melissa (lemon balm) or the citrus oils (see above) combined will make a sweet-smelling, sweat-beating blend.

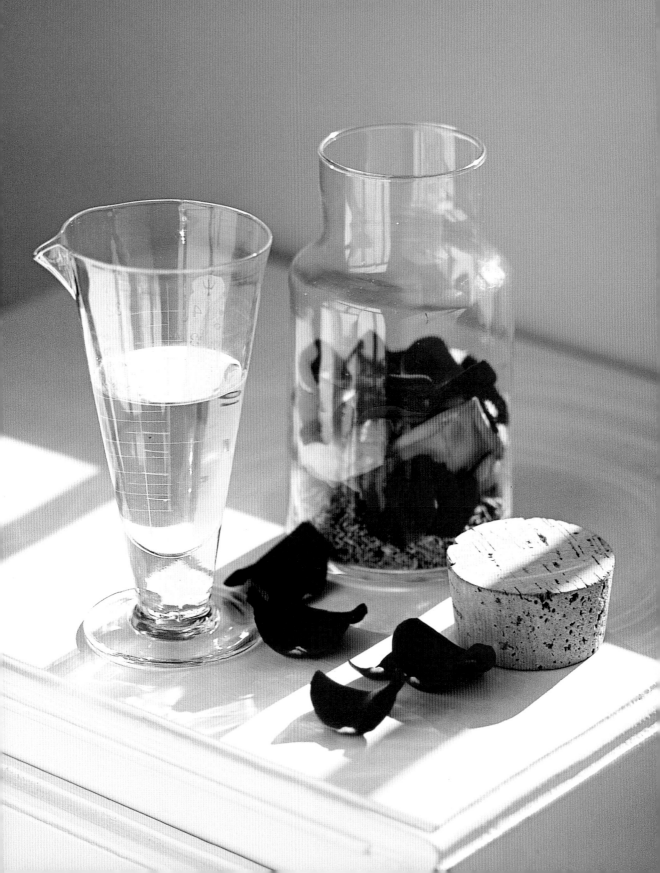

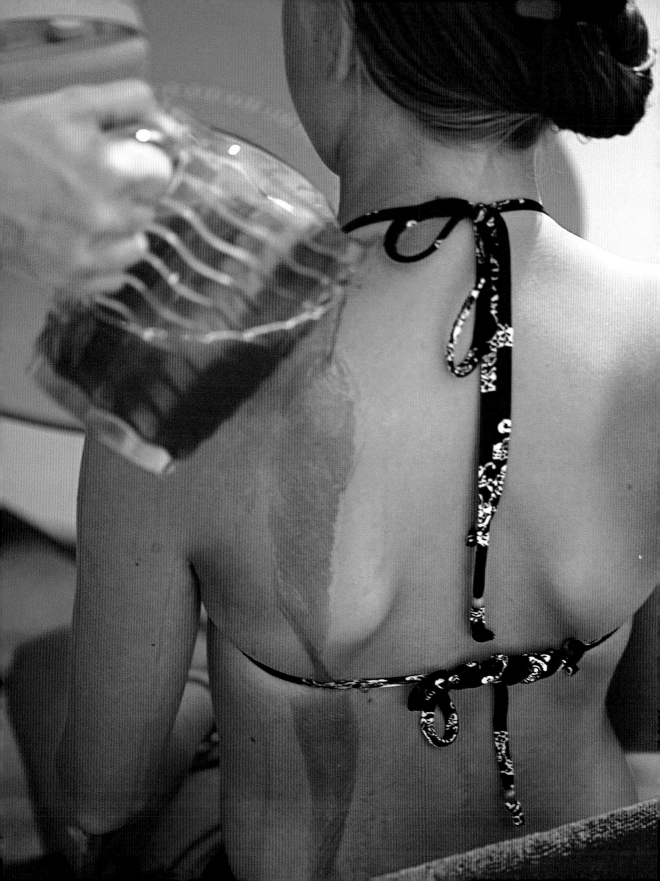

aloe vera after-sun soother

The gel in aloe vera leaves behind a gooey trail that is instantly both cooling and healing.

1 aloe vera leaf

This couldn't be simpler: just slice the aloe leaf in half and slide it slowly over the affected area. Repeat as often as you like.

mint and black tea sunburn solution

Used straight from the fridge, this takes the heat out of sunburn in a flash. And while we all know sunburn shouldn't happen – well, sometimes we all make mistakes…

110g (4oz) fresh mint leaves
3–4 black tea bags
1 litre (1³/4 pints) boiling water

Pour the boiling water over the mint and the teabags; cover, allow to stand for 10 minutes and strain. Cool, then transfer to a glass jar. Apply to sunburned skin using cotton wool pads. The tannic acid in the black tea draws the heat from the burn and restores the skin's acid balance, while the mint has an immediately cooling effect. This mixture keeps in the fridge for a few weeks.

more after-sun skin savers…

Smearing **yogurt** on your skin as soon as it turns pink can help unburn your sunburn, cooling your skin and re-establishing the vital pH balance, so it heals faster. Use plain, full-fat organic yogurt, if possible. Let it sit on your skin until it warms up, rinse with tepid water, then reapply. (Applying yogurt from the fridge is very soothing, too, taking the heat out of the area.)

Sunburn can also be cooled with **strawberries**: mash them and apply for 5 minutes to take the heat out of skin – or (even more effectively, on a face that's caught the sun), mash 1 tablespoon yogurt with 2 strawberries, and smooth onto the face. Instant relief.

Witch hazel, cucumber juice and cider vinegar all work to calm overheated skin: add 1 tablespoon of any of these to 225ml (8fl oz) water, put in a spritzer bottle and simply zoosh onto skin as required.

Although of course with sunburn, prevention is always better than cure…

I prefer not to use chemical sunscreens on my skin. Instead, I choose sun creams which are formulated using sun 'blocks' – mineral ingredients (titanium dioxide and zinc oxide), which 'bounce' light off the skin before it can trigger damage. Dr Hauschka and Liz Earle Naturally Active (see RESOURCES pp. 154–7) both make excellent sun ranges using natural mineral sunblocks, rather than chemical screens.

rosemary foot reviver

The mint and rosemary in this recipe are naturally cooling and invigorating, while the lactic acid in the milk is soothing. If you put pebbles or marbles in the bottom of the bowl, you can roll your toes over them while you soak your feet, which is totally relaxing for body, soul – and soles.

225ml (8fl oz) milk
50g (2oz) fresh mint leaves
6 large sprigs of fresh rosemary
6 drops peppermint essential oil

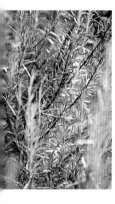

Put the milk and fresh herbs in a small pan over a low heat and simmer for 15 minutes. Remove the pan from the heat, and pour into a bowl large enough to bathe your feet in. Top up with warm or cool water, as preferred – or, best of all, some more milk. Add the peppermint essential oil, drop by drop, and swish.

no sweat foot spray

Cypress, rosemary and patchouli are all effective antibacterial and deodorant botanicals, and this spray will effectively help wipe out the odour-causing bacteria that thrive in the moist, warm environment they love best: your shoes…

2 sprigs rosemary
125ml (4fl oz) distilled witch hazel
35 drops cypress essential oil
5 drops patchouli essential oil

Put the sprigs of rosemary inside a spray bottle and add the other ingredients; shake well. Use it a couple of times a day, and carry it with you in summer (it can be spritzed through tights, if required).

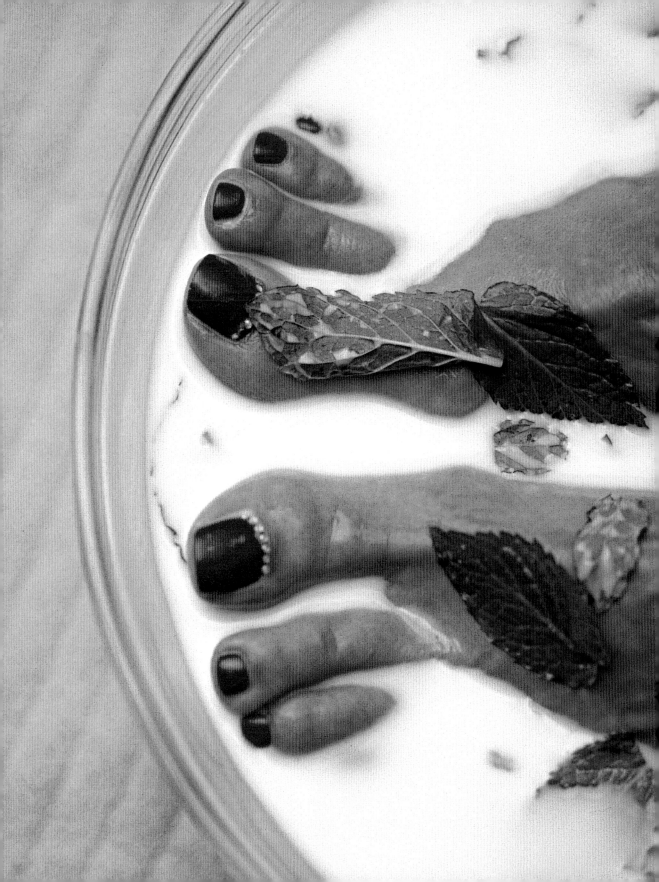

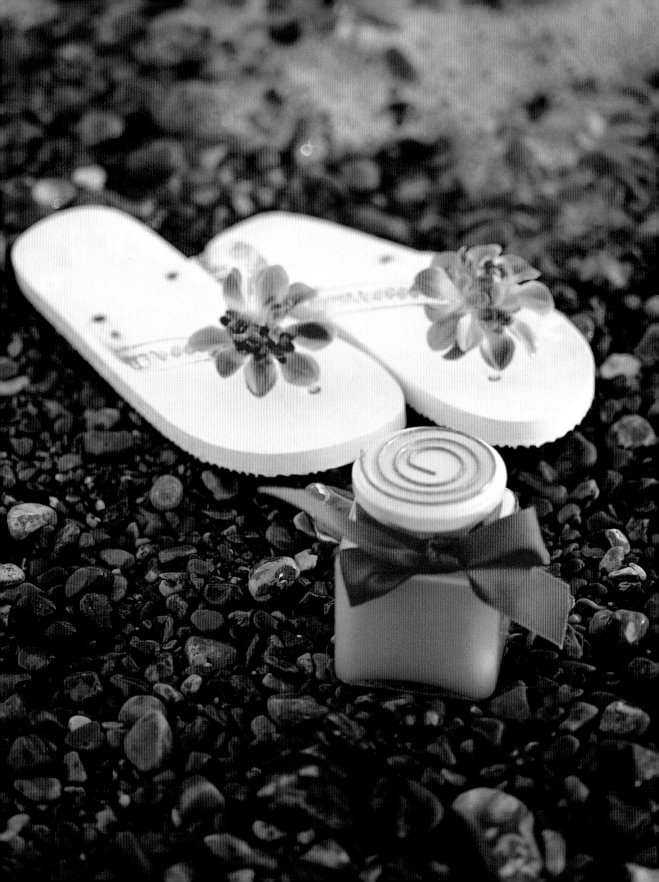

D.I.Y. foot bliss

• Ensure your feet are warm; soak for 5–15 minutes in a footbath of warm, not hot, water (or do the massage after a night-time bath). Towel dry before the massage.

• Sit in a comfortable chair with one leg crossed over the other and with the sole of one foot facing you.

• Move your thumbs over the raised foot in a circular fashion; get in and knead hard, without discomfort. Concentrating on a small area at a time, gradually work from your toes towards your heel, moving the fluids in your feet towards your heart. As you rub, pay extra attention to any area that feels 'crystallised' or knotty. Massaging these areas, in particular, helps dispel tension.

• Turn your foot over. Use your thumbs – more gently – to pull on the toes, and wiggle them side to side between thumb and forefinger.

• Switch feet and repeat the whole massage. Give it as much time as you can – in a perfect world, that would be 10–15 minutes, but if you can grab even 3 minutes (a minute and a half per foot) it will make a difference, in my experience.

peppermint foot balm

Use this balm at night for a rich, skin-softening foot massage; it's also incredible for smoothing rough skin on heels, ensuring feet are worthy of even the most elegant Manolo mules.

Petals from 24 calendula flowers (or 10 g/^{1}/$_2$fl oz dried flowers)
75ml (3fl oz) sweet almond oil
1 tablespoon avocado oil
20g (^{3}/$_4$oz) beeswax
40 drops peppermint essential oil

Put the calendula flowers in the bottom of a bottle and pour the oils over the top. Place in direct sunlight to speed up the infusion of the calendula into the oils. After 3 weeks, strain through a sieve – mashing the calendula to squeeze out the last of the goodness. Heat the beeswax in the oil in the top of a double-boiler until melted (see p.153). Remove from the heat and allow to cool slightly before adding the peppermint essential oil, drop by drop, and decanting into a sterilised jar. I use this every night after I've washed my feet and dried them thoroughly. (My Chinese herbalist told me that in China, foot-washing is a nightly ritual; the Chinese believe toxins and germs are excreted through the feet and it's important to sluice them away before going to bed so they can't be reabsorbed. All I can say is that I seem to get fewer colds and less 'flu than most people I know – and thanks to this balm, my feet are silky-soft.)

Feet also love...

Several other herbs will effectively help put the spring back in your step: make enough tea from the herbs (see p. 153) to comfortably cover your feet, and soak them in it while still warm. Try lavender as an instant tonic, horsetail for tired feet (and to reduce sweatiness), thyme for cleansing, or lovage as a strong natural deodorant.

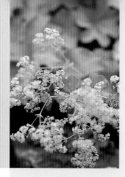

lady's mantle hand softener

Keep this soothing hand-softener in the fridge and apply daily – it's wonderful after washing up.

10g (¹/₂oz) fresh or 5g (¹/₄oz) dried lady's mantle leaves and flowers
10g (¹/₂oz) fresh or 5g (¹/₄oz) dried lemon balm leaves
150ml (¹/₄ pint) filtered, mineral or rainwater
50ml (2fl oz) lemon juice
30ml (1fl oz) vodka
4 drops sweet orange essential oil
4 tablespoons vegetable glycerine

Chop the lady's mantle and lemon balm and put in a pan with the water. Bring to the boil, simmer for 10 minutes and then allow to cool thoroughly; strain. Take 4 tablespoons of this infusion and pour into a sterilised bottle with a cork or a screw-top; add the other ingredients and seal. Shake well.

TIP

Face masks work wonders on hands, too – cleansing or delivering a moisture surge. Next time you indulge in one of the face masks in this book, slather it over your hands, too – then rest your hands on a towel for 10–15 minutes while it works its magic.

LADY'S MANTLE
Alchemilla mollis

Lady's mantle is decidedly unladylike in its promiscuity: it seeds itself between cracks and paving stones, and in the tiniest, most inhospitable crevices. That's why I love it. (HRH The Prince of Wales, meanwhile – a keen organic gardener – has it growing rampantly over his back terrace, and very pretty it looks, too.) It's the leaves of the plant you're after: they have astringent properties and according to herbal lore, will both heal pimples and keep wrinkles at bay. In northern climes, women have traditionally used a decoction (see p. 153) of lady's mantle for breast-firming (and I've put a recipe for this on p. 108). It's also reputed to be good for stopping bleeding from skin abrasions (gardeners, please note). The froth of tiny lime-green/yellow star-like flowers bloom for months. Gorgeous, gorgeous, gorgeous.

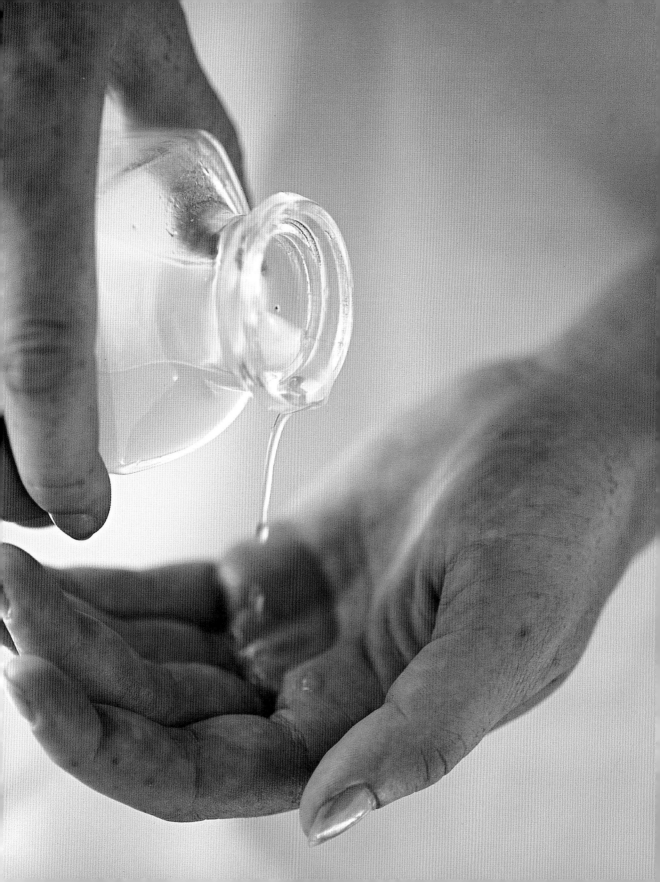

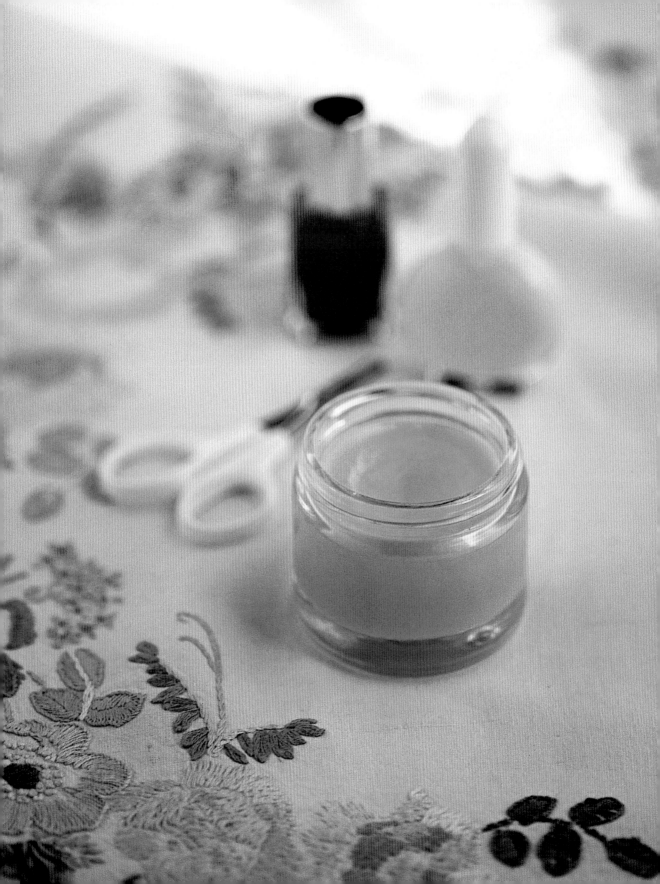

marsh mallow hand soother

MARSH MALLOW
Althaea officinalis

The Greeks and the Romans were big fans of marsh mallow, although it's said to have been used since prehistoric times. Its name comes from the Greek *altha*, 'to cure' – a clue to marsh mallow's healing and anti-inflammatory properties, which also make it a boon in cosmetics. The sugary roots produce mucilage – think sticky, gummy, viscous – which, blended into creams or lotions, is wonderfully skin-calming, soothing, softening and emollient. (Good for glossing hair, too, in conditioners.) It's said to control oily skin, help prevent breakouts – and to ease sensitivity. Typically, the dried roots – which you can harvest and dry yourself or buy from a herbalist – are made into a decoction (see p.153), although the fresh leaves can also be useful – as in the hand cream recipe.

This attractive shrub-like perennial (it's a relative of the hollyhock) has large grey-green leaves and clusters of pink flowers – but you'll need to lift it to get to the root, so grow enough to spare. It likes waterlogged ground, or to be kept damp. (Well, it is called 'marsh' mallow.)

This makes a fabulously smoothing, soothing barrier cream for housework or gardening – or replenishes natural moisture and velvetiness, whenever hands are dry and rough.

10g (½oz) marsh mallow leaves (fresh or dried)
200ml (7fl oz) still mineral water
10g (½oz) beeswax
10g (½oz) cocoa butter
50g (2oz) sweet almond oil
4 drops grapefruit seed extract
10 drops sweet orange essential oil
10 drops lemon essential oil

Put the marsh mallow leaves and the water in a pan, bring to the boil, then simmer for about 10 minutes. Remove from the heat and leave until lukewarm, then strain the mixture and measure off 40 ml (1½fl oz) of the liquid back into the pan. Heat the beeswax and cocoa butter in the oil in the top of a double-boiler until melted (see p. 153). Reheat the marsh mallow liquid until almost boiling and add it to the beeswax mixture, a little at a time. (The liquid has to be hot, otherwise the oils will set.) As you add the liquid, mix with a hand blender to create a creamy emulsion, and lastly add the grapefruit seed extract and essential oils, drop by drop. Put into dry, sterilised jars and seal. Any extra jars can be kept in the fridge to maintain freshness, but the jar in use won't need refrigerating.

nail and cuticle nourishing cream

Horsetail is best picked in spring, when it's flowering – but any time will do, and if you can't get fresh horsetail, dried is next best thing. Benzoin resin, meanwhile, is also ultra-nourishing for the cuticles and the nail bed, as well as being antiseptic and a natural preservative.

50g (2oz) fresh horsetail stems or
*   25g (1oz) dried horsetail*
150ml (1/4 pint) olive oil
1 tablespoon beeswax
10 drops vitamin E oil
5 drops benzoin resin
15 drops lavender essential oil (optional)

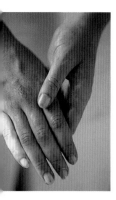

Pick the horsetail and lay it on a cloth to wilt overnight. Heat the horsetail in the oil in the top of a double-boiler (see p. 153) at a simmer for 30 minutes. Grate or chop the beeswax (unless you're using granules). Strain off the horsetail and return the oil to the double-boiler; add the beeswax and stir until melted. Remove from heat, and immediately add the benzoin resin and the vitamin E oil. (It's best to use a dropper for this.) Stir; pour into small jars and while it's still liquid, add the essential oil, drop by drop, and stir with a chopstick. Allow to cool thoroughly before sealing. Use nightly before bedtime for strong, flexible, snap-resistant nails.

nail booster oil

Horsetail is very rich in silica, which is a miraculous nail-strengthener (as well as other minerals like iron, magnesium and potassium), and after a few weeks' use your nails should be strong and flexible – the ideal combination. (You don't want nails so hard that they snap – which is the effect most commercial nail hardeners have.)

20g (3/4oz) fresh horsetail stems or
*   10g (1/2oz) dried horsetail, finely chopped*
2 tablespoons sweet almond oil – or, better still,
*   neem oil (I use Neal's Yard Remedies)*

Place the horsetail and the oil in the top of a double-boiler (see p. 153) and heat gently. Allow to cool and pour the whole mixture into a screw-top jar; leave to stand for 1 week in the sun, then strain the oil. Use this nightly, ideally on unvarnished nails, and massage into cuticles, to stimulate blood flow. For a deep nail-strengthening treatment, once a week gently warm this oil in a double-boiler and soak nails for 20 minutes. You can reuse it time and again; just pour back into the bottle.

TIP

To whiten nails – particularly if they have gone yellow from the use of polish – mix 1 teaspoon lemon juice into 1 tablespoon orangeflower water. Keep in a clean, sealable container and once a day, soak a cotton wool pad in the mixture; sweep over nails. Moisturise your hands and cuticles afterwards.

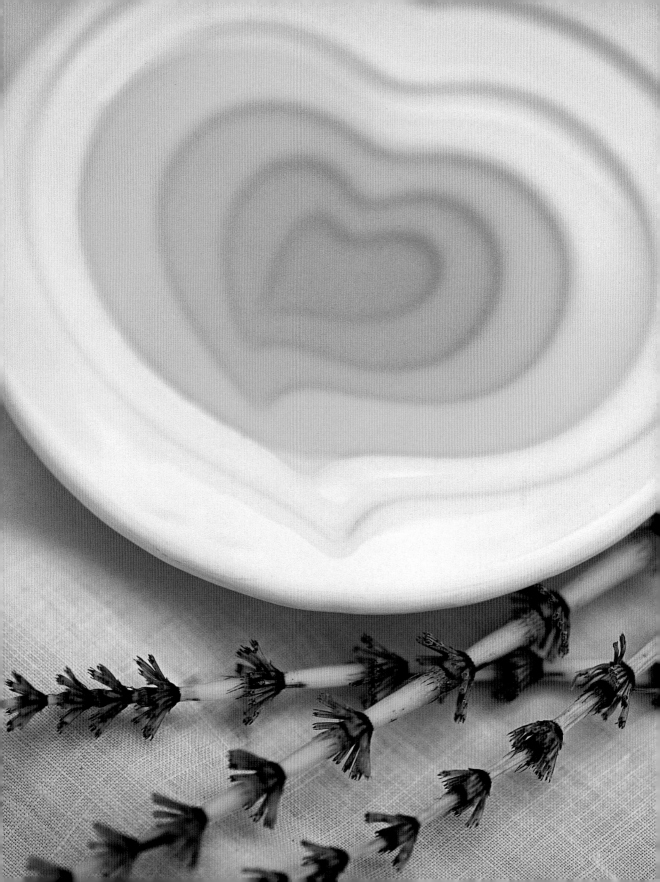

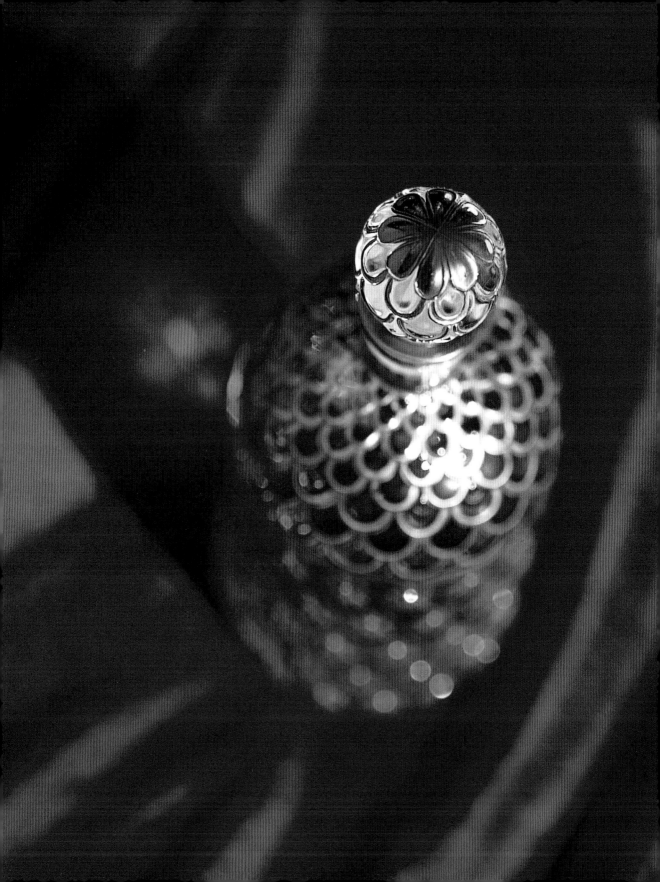

ravishing rose cologne

Alcohol is wonderful for extracting the fragrance from plants – as ancient perfumers knew. (And it's very sterile, ensuring that home-made colognes and scents don't go 'off'.) Alcohol is, in fact, still the main ingredient of most contemporary fragrances. Tincture of benzoin has a vanilla-like fragrance.

110g (4oz) fresh, scented rose petals (which must
*   be unsprayed)*
600ml (1 pint) vodka
50 drops rose essential oil
15 drops geranium essential oil
10 drops tincture of benzoin
50ml (2fl oz) vegetable glycerine

Put the rose petals in a large glass container. Put the vodka in a separate jug, and add the essential oils, drop by drop, the tincture of benzoin and, lastly, the glycerine. Pour over the rose petals. Shake daily for 3 weeks and decant into a beautiful bottle.

sun-ripened tomato cologne

A few years ago, my friends at the Demeter fragrance company in the USA brought out a 'green tomato cologne', which was a huge success. I love the smell of tomato leaves, which always remind me of my grandfather's conservatory. This is a summery, unisex cologne.

25g (1oz) fresh tomato leaves
Zest of 1 medium-sized lemon
1 teaspoon chopped fresh basil leaves
225ml (8fl oz) vodka
10 drops juniper essential oil
1/2 teaspoon vegetable glycerine

Chop the tomato leaves and the lemon zest. Put in the bottom of a sterilised jar or bottle with the basil; add the vodka and the juniper essential oil, drop by drop. Hide it in a cool, dark place for 2–3 weeks – but try to remember to shake it occasionally. Strain the liquid through muslin (or kitchen paper), add the glycerine and pour into a bottle with a cork or screw-top. Splash and spray as much as you like.

Once you've experimented with the fragrances on these few pages, try similar recipes using the leaves and flowers of plants you love, to create your own 'signature' scent, experimenting with essential oils to turbo-charge the fragrance.

hungary water

Splash or spritz this all over for instant freshness and fragrance.

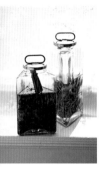

25g (1oz) fresh lemon balm leaves or
* 1 tablespoon of dried lemon balm*
50g (2oz) fresh rosemary leaves
1 fresh mint sprig (only use fresh –
* omit if you don't have any)*
Thinly pared rind of ¹/₂ a lemon
300ml (¹/₂ pint) vodka
125ml (4fl oz) orangeflower water
125ml (4fl oz) rosewater

Chop the lemon balm and put all the herbs and the lemon rind in the bottom of a glass jar. Add the vodka, cover tightly and shake well. Leave in a warm place – or on a windowsill – for 3 weeks, remembering to shake it every day. Then strain and, as a last step, add the orangeflower and rosewater. Decant into a sterilised bottle and use within 6 months.

The other way to extract fragrance is using by oil. Place your flowers in a jar – lilac, rose or jasmine all work well – and add enough extra virgin olive oil to cover. Shake it daily. After 2 weeks, strain the flowers through a sieve, pressing down to extract the last of the fragrant oils. You can use these subtly but beautifully perfumed oil in any of the recipes that call for olive oil – or simply massage into your pulse points and enjoy the subtle, powdery fragrance.

carmelite water

This was originally invented by Carmelite monks, as long ago as 1611. (Hence the name – although they knew it as 'Eau de Carmes'.) The monks created it as a money-spinner to keep the finances of the monastery healthy. This captures the sunny scent of lemon balm – which, at the time, was very fashionable in perfumes worn by royalty and the wealthy. Carmelite water was also taken internally, as a tonic – though don't try this at home!

50g (2oz) fresh angelica leaves
50g (2oz) fresh lemon balm leaves or
* 2 tablespoons of dried lemon balm*
10g (¹/₂oz) coriander seeds
1 heaped teaspoon freshly grated nutmeg
10g (¹/₂oz) cloves
2 x 5 cm (2 inch) cinnamon sticks
300ml (¹/₂ pint) vodka

This couldn't be easier: put the herbs and spices in the bottom of a glass jar, cover with the vodka and seal. Leave in a warm place – a windowsill is fine – and shake the bottle every day for 3–4 weeks. Strain into a sterilised bottle with a cork or screw-top and – like the Hungary water – use within 6 months.

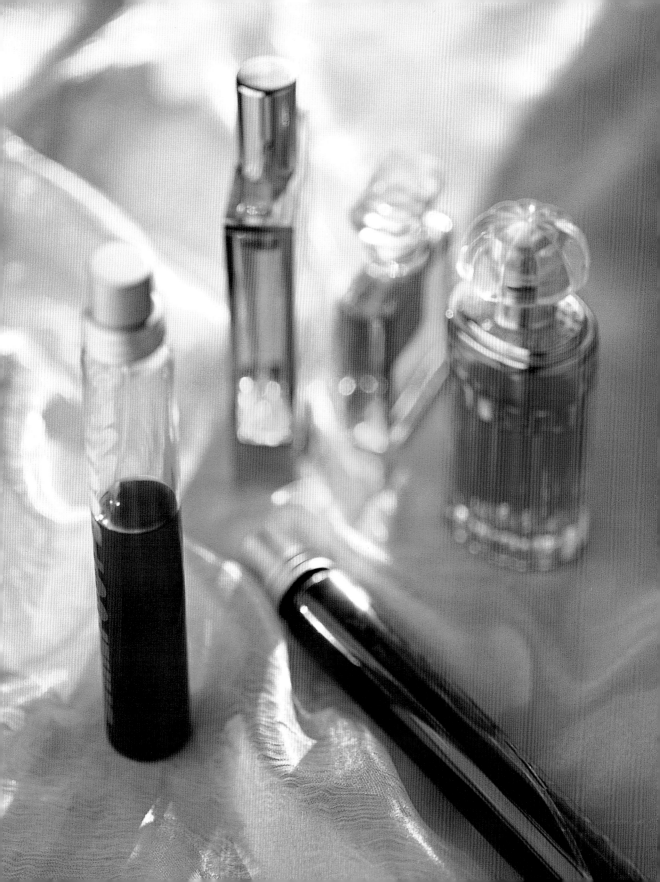

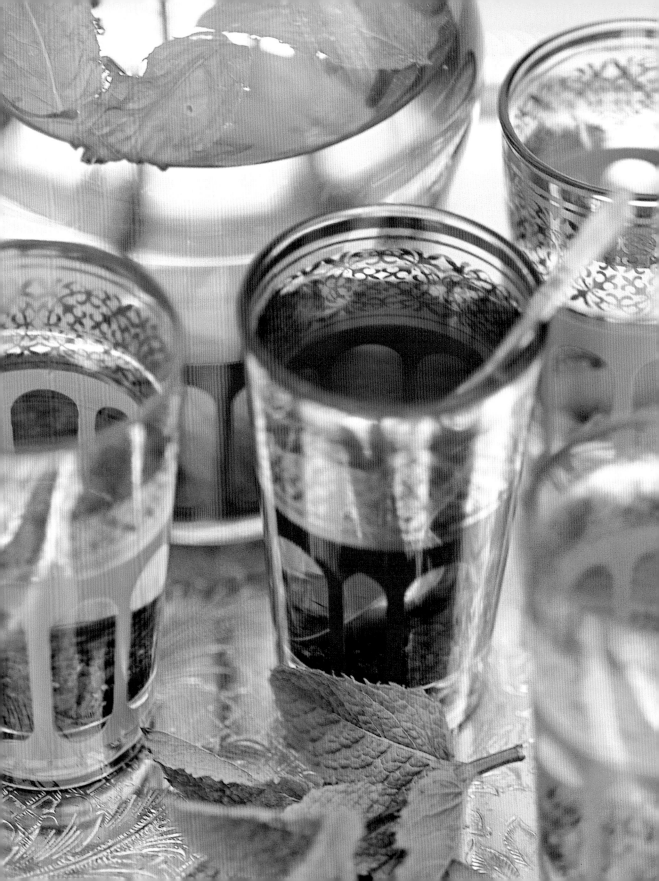

teas your skin and hair will love...

Put the kettle on. Because true radiance comes not just from what you put on your face, body and hair, but what you eat and drink and how you feel. A varied, wholesome (and preferably organic) diet will work wonders – but if you want to look gorgeous, discover the beauty power of herbal teas, enjoyed in place of caffeine...

birch tea

Recommended for sluggish circulation, spots or dull skin. Ideally, use young fresh or dried birch leaves; or you can buy dried birch leaves from herbalists. To make the tea, steep 12 fresh leaves (or 1 teaspoon dried ones) – in 225ml (8fl oz) boiling water for 8 minutes; add honey to taste. This creates a pleasant green, woody-flavoured tea which – for optimum results – should be enjoyed 3 times a day.

linden

Linden – also called lime blossom, or vervaine – is one of the best-known and loved herbs for tea. It's good for helping to keep freckles and wrinkles at bay. It's also supposed to stimulate hair growth – and, as a triple-whammy, calms the nerves and promotes sleep. To make the tea, gather the flowers when they smell strongly of honey. (Dried flowers can also be used, but once the scent fades, they're past their best.) You can also, of course, buy linden tea bags in natural food stores. The taste is a little chamomile-like: sweet, aromatic and appley. To make the tea, steep 2 teaspoons fresh flowers (or 1 teaspoon dried) in 225ml (8fl oz) boiling water for up to 10 minutes; add honey to taste if you have a sweet tooth.

rosehip tea

Sweet-smelling tea can be made from the petals and rosehips of most varieties – or you can buy rosehip tea commercially (and organically). The hips have high concentrations of vitamins A, B, E, K, P and especially C – and a cup of rosehips (that's the hips, not the tea) is said to contain as much vitamin C as 150 oranges. Vitamin C, in turn, is a powerful antioxidant, and thirst-quenching rosehip tea is a wonderful way to keep your reserves topped up. (Antioxidants help protect skin against free radical damage caused by smoke, pollution and sun damage.) If you harvest your own rosehips, grind the dried hips into a powder (using a pestle and mortar or a herb grinder), and use 1 teaspoon in 225ml (8fl oz) boiling water. Steep for about 5 minutes, and add a little honey. (This tea is good hot or cold.)

caraway tea

The Ancient Greeks prescribed caraway tea for pale young girls, to put a flush in their cheeks. (So if you're feeling run down or pasty, try this.) Grind or crush 1 teaspoon caraway seeds and cover with 225ml (8fl oz) boiling water. Steep to taste and sweeten if you like with honey.

facial booster massage

I swear by facial massage. Unlike some people – who are scared to touch their faces, anxious that too much movement leads to wrinkling – I'm convinced, instead, that facial massage improves the flow of oxygen to the skin, boosts collagen and elastin production, keeps the lymph flowing (so dispelling toxins), and ensures skin glows beautifully, as well as reducing facial tension. (What more could you ask?) So every night, using a facial oil, I follow this technique. Apply your cleansing cream or an oil, and do the same. I'm sure you'll see a difference, if you do it regularly.

  Use your middle (longest) finger for the massage. Do both sides of the face at once (mirroring the movements), except for a few points in the centre of the face for which you should use either your right or left hand. In a perfect world, you'd stimulate each point for 1 minute. In reality, 5–10 seconds on each point can still make a difference. Don't move your fingers over the skin; move the face itself, with your fingers.

1 Find the spot at the hairline that's directly above the centre of the eye. Massage using inward circles.

2 Move fingers down the face to half-way between eyebrows and hairline. Massage using inward circles.

3 This spot uses your thumbs: locate the spot on either side of the bridge of the nose, just below the browline. Push upwards, using pressure rather than circling technique. (NB This can hurt!)

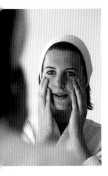

4 At the outer tip of the eyebrows, massage with outward circles.

5 At the outside corner of the eyes, gently massage outwards.

6 On the top of the cheekbone, underneath the middle of the eye, circle outwards.

7 Now move the fingers down until they are in line with your nostrils (roughly the apple of the cheek), and massage using outward circles.

8 In the indentation that runs from the middle of your nose to your top lip, circle in a clockwise direction (one finger only).

9 Locate the middle of your chin (where a 'dimple' would be), and again, massage in clockwise circles (one finger only).

10 Using both fingers again, place fingers on the jawline either side of the chin. Circle outwards.

11 Move fingers outwards along the jaw to a point mid-way between jaw and the jaw-hinge. Massage in outward circles.

12 Find the muscle just in front of the jaw hinge – where there is a slight indentation. With the mouth resting open, massage in circles towards the back of your head.

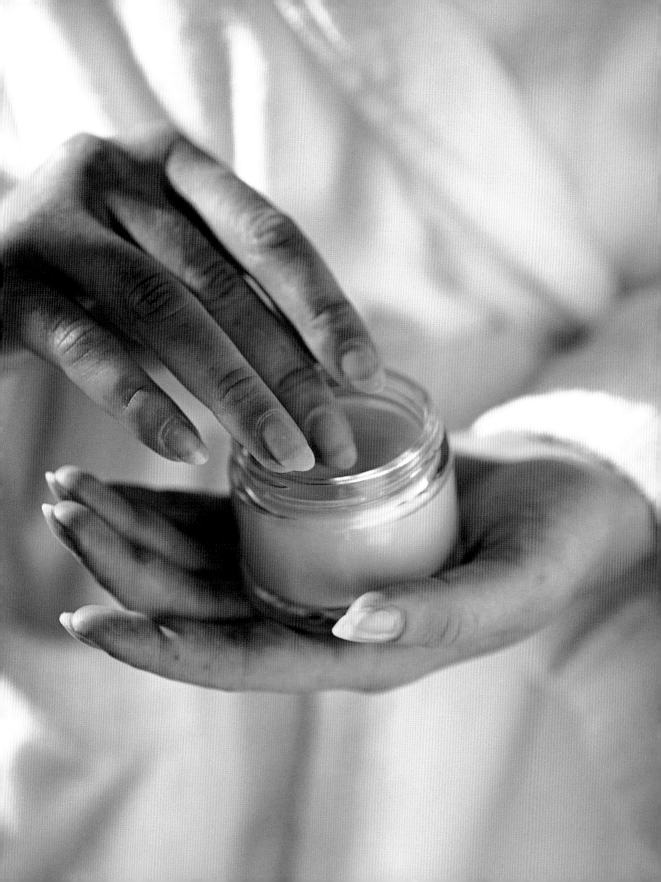

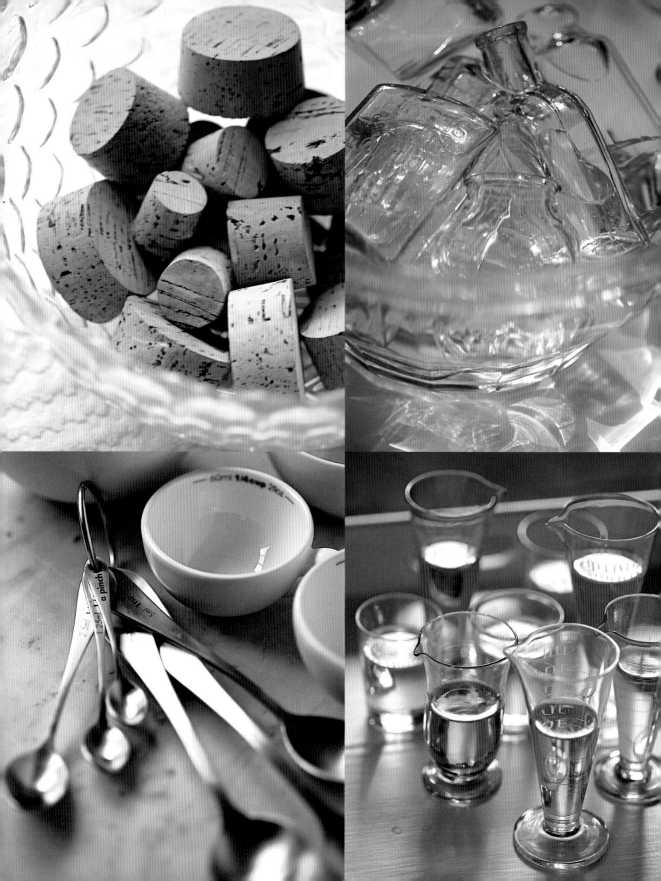

how to...

So: now you've read the recipes. Decided to become **a natural beauty**. But before you start, you need to know the basics. This section is **the nitty-gritty**: equipment you'll need, simple techniques, a few **precautions** to ensure that your cosmetics are **safe** and **sterile**. Plus, you'll discover lots more **store cupboard and botanical ingredients** – and what they can do for you and your skin. It's not the sexiest bit of the book, which is why I put it at the back. But it is a must-read. (Anyway, who reads books from start to finish these days?) And once you've mastered what's in these pages, you're not just ready to follow my recipes – but to start experimenting with your own...

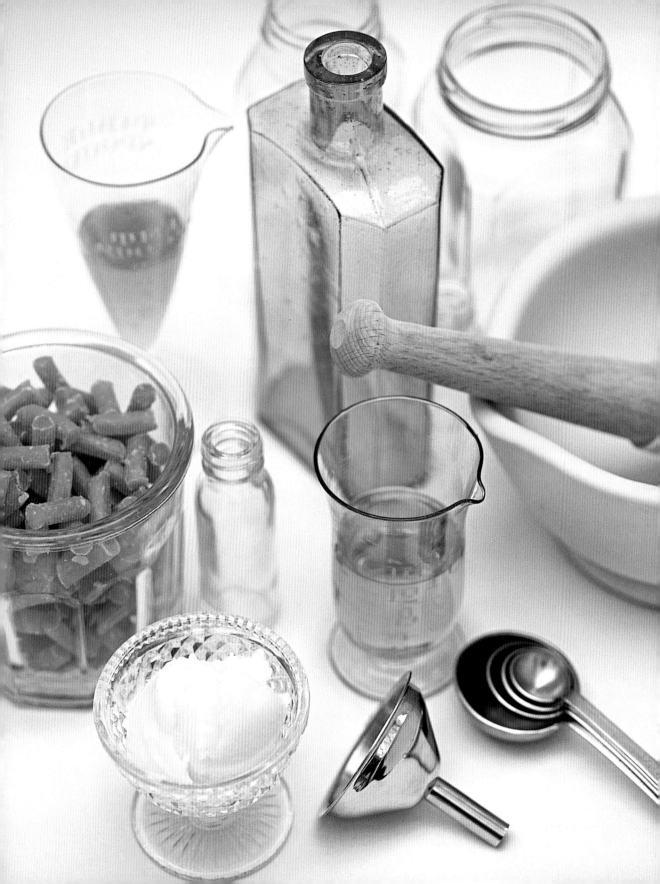

essential equipment

As I said at the start of this book, if you can make a vinaigrette dressing or melt chocolate, you can make cosmetics. You don't really need any special equipment: your regular kitchen gear is perfectly adequate. (You'll certainly find most of this list in the average, well-stocked kitchen.) But it does help, I find, to be organised. Ideally, you should have to hand the following equipment – though you certainly won't need everything for every recipe. (If a chef's equipment is his *batterie de cuisine*, think of this as your *batterie de beauté*...)

• Kettle

• Heat-resistant jugs (if you use glass, make sure it's Pyrex, or similarly heatproof)

• Heat-resistant bowls (see above)

• Stainless steel or enamel pans (aluminium can stain, and there's a health question mark over it)

• A double-boiler or *bain marie* – probably the most-used item among my cosmetic-making equipment

• Measuring scales (I use electronic scales but this is largely a matter of preference, though they're great for measuring tiny amounts)

• Measuring spoons (I like Nigella Lawson's, which clip and unclip)

• Measuring cups (again, Nigella Lawson's – are gorgeous, and usefully feature imperial, metric and US cup equivalents)

• I also use a Taler metal measuring jug marked with quantities and volumes of different liquids and solids, and find this very handy (easier than using the scales all the time, although probably not quite so precise)

• Herb or coffee grinder

• Food processor or blender (I use a Magimix)

• Pestle and mortar

• Hand whisk or hand blender (I use a Braun)

• Wooden and metal spoons for stirring

• Sharp knives for cutting

• A vegetable peeler (I swear by GoodGrips)

• A grater (and a Microplane is an asset)

• A large sieve and smaller, mesh tea strainer

• Muslin – or plenty of kitchen paper (which I find works just as well) for straining

• Sterilised bottles, jars and plastic containers in which to store and display your finished products

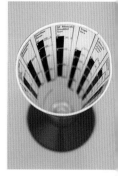

• A selection of different sizes of large glass containers in which to infuses oils and alcohol-based liquids like fragrances and deodorants; these needn't be expensive and I look for them at car boot sales and in thrift stores (mine are old sweetie jars I picked up for a song)

When you're making cosmetics, clear the workspace of any food before you start. Make sure you've got plenty of elbow room, and heatproof surfaces on which to place pans or hot jugs. (Bread boards or trivets are ideal.) I find it easiest to lay out everything I'm going to need – including any pre-grated, cleaned or sliced ingredients – so it's all to hand.

storing and packaging your cosmetics

I'm as much of a sucker for gorgeous packaging as the next person. (Frankly, I'm almost physically incapable of throwing away anything with the double-C Chanel logo on it!) And one of the

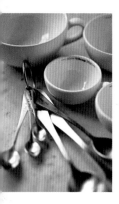

downsides of natural and organic cosmetics that you could buy in the stores, until recently, was that the packaging was often off-puttingly hideous. I didn't really want it on my bathroom shelf, and it didn't seduce me into wanting to use it.

When I make my own cosmetics, I want to get sensual pleasure out of the ritual of using them. So, to maximise the enjoyment you get out of yours, I do recommend you package them as gorgeously as you can. Save jars and bottles and small tins that you like, and clean them thoroughly after use, soaking off any labels. Great sources for jars and bottles, in my experience, are thrift stores, charity shops, car boot sales, antique emporia and junk shops, as well as kitchen equipment stores and mail order catalogues. Once you've 'got your eye in' you'll see potential packaging for your creams and lotions in all sorts of places.

The snag is that often, they don't have a lid or stopper – but to my mind, that's what corks are for. I am lucky enough to live near one of those wonderful old-fashioned hardware stores (Butler's Emporium in Hastings Old Town deserves a name-check here), which still has brooms and clothes airers hanging from the ceiling – and a huge stock of different-sized corks, with one to fit almost every container. If you aren't lucky enough to have a Butler's Emporium on your doorstep, have a snoop round hardware stores when you're travelling – at home and abroad. (Continental Europe, in particular, is still a treasure-trove of these places. I've brought corks back from Spain, Italy and France; sad but true. Still, as souvenirs go, they're very lightweight and don't take up much suitcase space!)

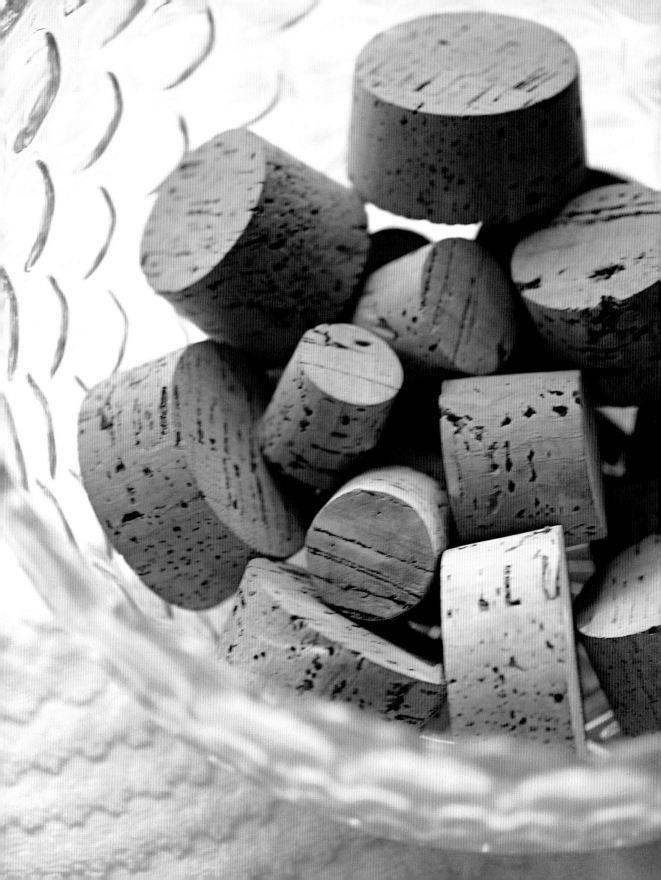

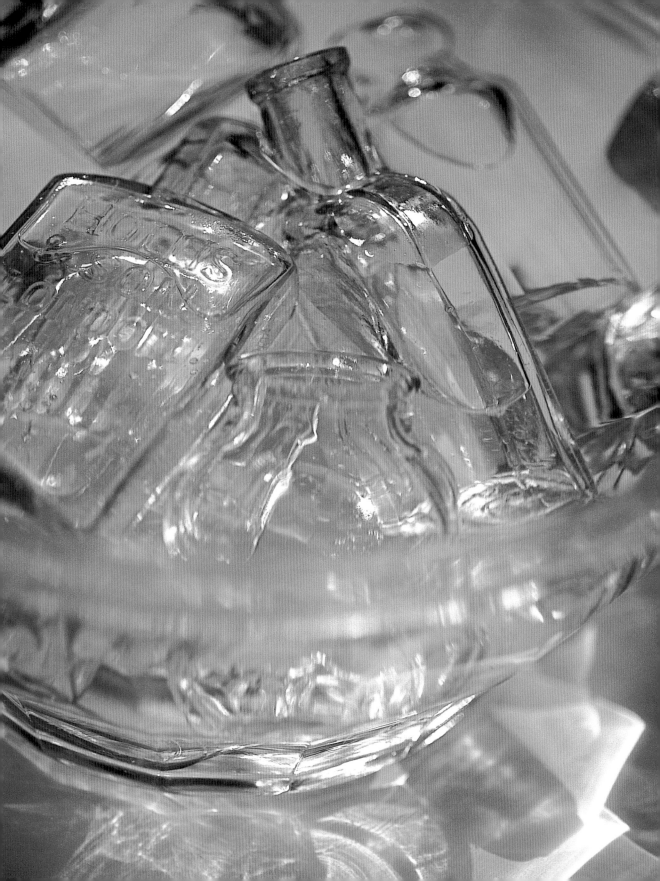

play it safe

Home-made cosmetics have no preservatives to give them an almost indefinite shelf-life (unlike the ones you buy in a beauty hall or pharmacy). So it pays to follow some simple precautions that will maximise their shelf-life and prevent them going 'off', or becoming contaminated in any way.

• Your storage jars or bottles must be perfectly sterile. First, scrub them carefully, including all the crevices or rims, using a washing-up liquid. (Bottle brushes of different sizes are very handy for this.) I prefer to use an ecological washing-up liquid, like Ecover, since for me this is all about keeping things as natural and chemical-free as possible.

• Sterilise glass jars or metal containers: either wash well in soapy water then place in a warm oven 130°C/250°F/gas ½ for 30 minutes, or wash as above, and boil the jars in a large pan, covered with water, for 15 minutes. (Lids and tops too.) Dry with a fresh, clean cloth and upturn them onto another clean cloth until used, so they can't trap dust or dirt inside. For plastic containers: first establish they're heatproof, place in a large pan, cover with water and bring slowly to the boil. Boil for 2–3 minutes and lift them out with tongs. Allow to drain and then dry with a fresh, clean cloth.

• It's vital to allow your cosmetics to cool properly before sealing them, otherwise you risk contamination from condensation. Also, replace lids, screw-tops or corks after using something. This keeps bugs out – helping to preserve the life of your beauty products.

• Always follow the storage guidelines. If something needs to be kept in the fridge, do just that, and always discard when it starts to smell 'off' or the texture changes. (If the colour fades, that's less of a clue, as that tends to happen naturally and isn't in itself harmful.)

how to do a patch test

You need to carry out a patch test before applying products to your face or large areas of the body. Apply a small amount of the potion to your inner arm, just below the elbow, or behind one ear. Cover with sticking plaster (unless you're allergic to it), and leave for 24 hours. If there is any soreness, redness or irritation, your skin is reacting to an ingredient and you should not use the product on a wider scale.

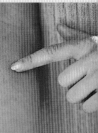

• Always wash your hands before using home-made cosmetics – actually, this is just plain common sense with all cosmetics, in order to avoid transferring any bacteria from your hands to your face, mouth or eyes.

• Never, ever share any cosmetics, not only your home-made ones. (If your partner or children swipe your skin cream, make them a jar of their own!)

FACT: all home-made cosmetics will keep for longer in a fridge – but you really needn't bother, with oil-and-beeswax mixtures or plain oil blends. There is a much bigger risk of contamination in products that contain water; bugs breed readily in water, but not in oils.

drying and storing herbs

Herbs – as wise women have always known – offer a natural beauty solution to most skin challenges, from oiliness to premature ageing. They provide gentle, organic nutrients and treatment for skin – because they're packed with minerals, chlorophyll and general concentrated plant goodness. When they're infused into oil or water, this herbal magic can then be absorbed into the skin. When herbs are dried, meanwhile, their goodness is concentrated – which is why most of the recipes in this book call for half the quantity of dried herbs as fresh. Ideally, you should use fresh herbs wherever possible. But this isn't practical year-round, in every climate. If you grow your own herbs, then, it's good to know how to preserve them…

Air drying is the most widely used method of drying herbs, but it must be done in a dry, well-ventilated room that's free from fumes and dust, and ideally somewhere the temperature can be maintained at 20–32°C (68–90°F). Speed is everything: if herbs take too long to dry, they can start to go mouldy or blacken – in which case they're useless. Hang the herbs upside down in small bunches using string or raffia (or ribbon looks pretty – see opposite).

Food dehydrators are a foolproof way of drying herbs, but take up quite a lot of space and are only really worth the investment if you're planning to harvest and dry large quantities.

Freezing herbs works really well: simply pack them in plastic bags when fresh and stick straight in the deep freeze. (Be sure to label the bag – it's amazing how every single herb looks the same once frozen!) Allow to thaw and then pat dry; use the quantity of fresh herbs specified in the recipe, not dried.

Oven drying is recommended for roots and woody plants which would take too long to dry if air-dried. Cut the roots crossways into thin slices or small pieces with a sharp knife. (This, I've found, is easier when they're still fresh.) Spread the cleaned and (towel) dried roots out on a baking sheet and dry them in the oven at the lowest setting possible. Keep an eye on them; the roots or stems should be dry within 2–3 hours. Leave to cool thoroughly.

Storing dried herbs and plants correctly is a must. When dried, the herbs should be packed in tightly sealed jars and labelled. (Put the date on the label somewhere so you know when you harvested them; fresh herbs are best and always throw out last year's harvest when this year's is in.) Choose small containers that exclude as much air as possible, as if there's too much air in the tin or jar, herbs can absorb moisture and go mouldy; lady's mantle and marsh mallow are particularly vulnerable to this.

NB If you buy dried herbs, buy organic – non-organic herbs are sometimes irradiated.

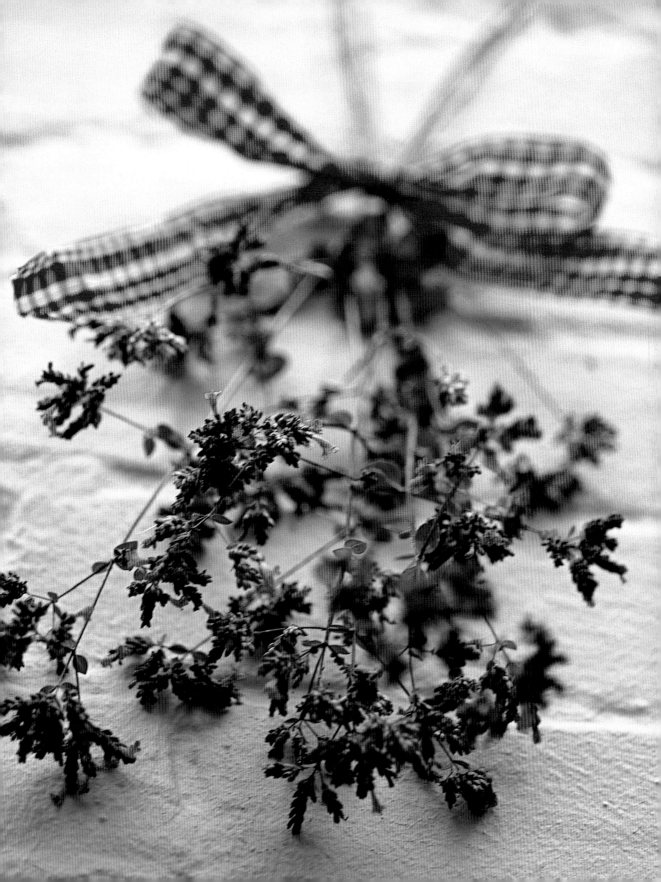

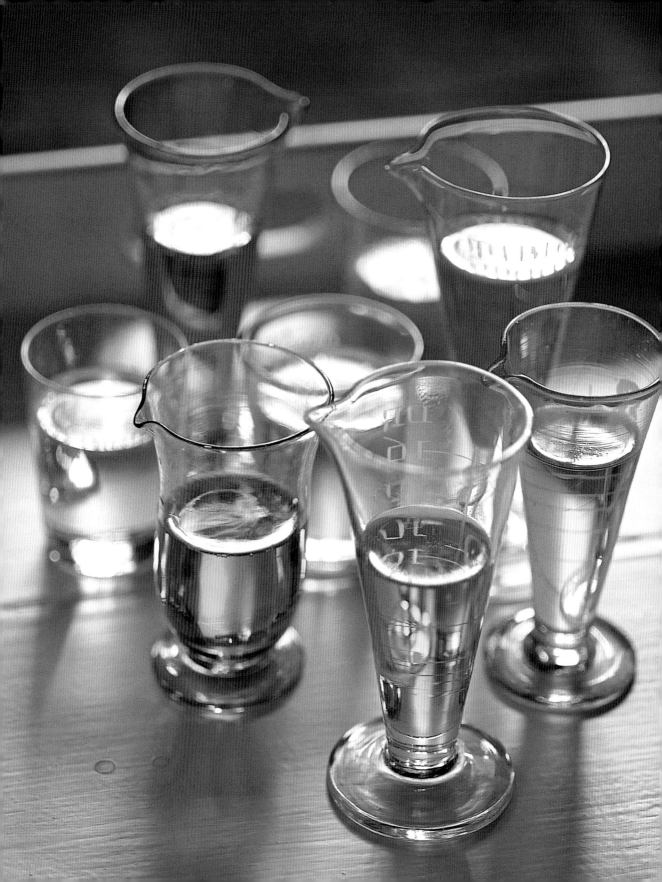

fabulous cosmetic oils

Plant oils are very skin-compatible – far more so than mineral oil (*Liquidum paraffinum*), a cheap and widely used ingredient in conventional cosmetics, which just sits on the skin's surface. The oils sink into skin, delivering nourishment and helping to protect the skin's 'barrier function', enabling skin to retain water and stay plumped-up and moisturised.

Different oils, though, have different properties. Once you've mastered the simple basics of making a few creams (melting beeswax into the oils – in the right quantity – basically turns them into a cream), you can experiment with your own combination of oils. Many of the following can be found in natural food stores or supermarkets; some you may have to source through a supplier (Neal's Yard Remedies offers the widest selection of organic oils that I've found).

WARNING
Nut oil sensitivity is becoming far more widespread; if you know you are allergic or sensitive to nuts (or there is a history of nut allergy in your family), you may also suffer a reaction if you put nut oils on your skin.

Almond oil or **sweet almond oil**; this pale yellow oil is pressed or expelled from nuts of the sweet almond tree. It's nourishing and blissfully skin-softening, and packed with vitamin E.

Apricot kernel oil A lightweight oil – from apricot stones – that sinks in fast, making it ideal for body treatments.

Argan oil There's a bit of a 'beauty buzz' about this oil, from the Moroccan argan tree; the locals use it as a hair pomade, massage oil – and for healing scar tissue and sun-damaged skin. Now it's emerging that argan is effective at neutralising free radical damage, which can lead to premature ageing. Try it in recipes that call for almond or avocado oil.

Avocado oil This pale green oil, which is compatible with most skintypes, is packed with betacarotene and vitamins C and E – and recent research shows it helps absorb UV radiation from the sun. (Though it won't take the place of sunscreen.)

Coconut oil This is sometimes solid at room temperature, but liquifies when heated (or in a warm environment). It creates a great barrier on skin – use a simple slick as a lip balm – and naturally locks in moisture. Try adding it to hair masks, if you have dry hair, or as the base for a massage oil.

Jojoba oil This is sometimes referred to as 'jojoba wax' (say it *ho-ho-ba*), but in fact it's a fairly viscous oil derived from the jojoba bean. Its composition is very like the skin's own sebum, making it highly skin-compatible. It gives creams a firm texture – but melts beautifully into skin at body temperature.

Olive oil Organic olive oil is my personal favourite all-round beauty multi-tasker. Pure skin magic: packed with polyphenol antioxidants (which help undo the free radical damage from sun and pollution exposure), nourishing, but not as quickly-absorbed as some oils. It's even used in some hospitals to treat rough, scaly skin, because of its skin-smoothing power. Olive oils should be cold-pressed extra virgin – and do go for organic, always.

Sunflower oil Sunflower oil, like jojoba, mirrors the skin's natural lipids – so it is good in skincare, as well as for massage blends; it's also a great hair conditioner and is ideal for 'macerating' herbs (see p. 112) to extract their goodness. (But buy a cosmetic quality, rather than the cooking variety you'll find on the grocery shelf.)

Wheatgerm oil This lightweight, nutty oil is quite strongly scented so I prefer to use it in small quantities to help 'preserve' cosmetics as it's rich in antioxidant vitamin E as well as vitamin B complex. Dry skins, though, lap it up, and I've even heard good reports from some eczema sufferers about wheatgerm oil's healing powers – although not everyone loves the slightly sour smell.

more wonders of the natural (beauty) world

Avocados These are packed with protein and natural oils, and rich in vitamins A and B. In some countries, women just mash avocado straight onto their skin or hair, for protection.

Beeswax Melted into oils, beeswax miraculously solidifies them, turning any oil into an easy-to-use cream. Beeswax is produced by bees to build the walls of their cells. It's non-pore-clogging, so it's suitable even for problem or oily skins.

Beer Beer – especially flat beer – makes a terrific setting lotion, and the sugar and protein combine to thicken hair and give it body. (You won't smell like an old pub: the smell disappears as soon as your hair dries.) Naturally, I'd recommend organic beer as most commercial beers contain chemical additives.

Bicarbonate of soda (baking soda) This can be the basis of a tooth powder – or be used in baths as a soothing soak for itchy skin. Try it in a footbath, to relax and to neutralise odour-causing bacteria and natural acids.

Borax Borax is a natural preservative, but is used to add texture to creams or body lotions. It soothes irritated skin, too.

Cider vinegar (sometimes spelled 'cyder vinegar') Made by fermenting natural apple juice, this is packed with minerals – think magnesium, calcium, iron and phosphorus – and very skin-friendly. (In fact, used in bath water or toners, cider vinegar helps restore skin's acid balance.)

Cocoa butter Skins love this: it melts at body temperature and is wonderfully lubricating and smoothing. A great barrier to lock in moisture.

Cornflour (or cornstarch) This is made from powdered maize kernels, and a perfect alternative to talc. (It eases irritated skin, too.)

Fuller's earth A type of clay sold as a fine, grey powder. It makes a great base for masks and hair packs, blended with other ingredients.

Glycerine What's known as a 'humectant', glycerine attracts moisture to the skin, and gives creams and lotions a nice 'slip'. Be sure to source plant-derived glycerine – for example, from Neal's Yard Remedies – as a lot of glycerine today is a by-product of the petroleum industry.

Honey Honey is a versatile, multi-purpose ingredient: it's antiseptic, astringent – but moisturising, too. (Look out for Manuka honey, from New Zealand, which can be used as a treatment for break-outs, simply smeared on skin and washed off again, because of its antibacterial action.)

Kaolin A fine, white, powdered clay, kaolin can be used in masks and body packs to draw impurities from the skin.

Lemon juice Lemon juice is naturally astringent and works as a mild alternative to bleach. It's good on stained nails; a little harsh for hair.

Oatmeal Soothing and gentle, oatmeal makes a fantastic bath additive. Dry, irritated skins love it – and it's miraculous on rashes or skin abrasions. It's very cleansing – and a handful of oats can even be used in place of soap.

Rosewater Rosewater and orangeflower water are skin-soothing by-products of the manufacture of essential oils, created by steam distillation. Orangeflower water can be substituted in most recipes that call for rosewater. If you prefer the scent of neroli to roses, use this instead.

Shea butter Richly nourishing, shea butter (also known as karité butter) makes for smooth and supple skin; it's a great base for creams and lotions, but can also be slathered on skin on its own, for instant silkiness.

Tincture of benzoin Benzoin is actually a resin from the benzoin tree (*Styrax benzoin*), used as a fixative in perfumes and pot pourris; it also has a naturally preservative action. You only need a few drops.

Witch hazel This clear lotion is distilled from the bark and twigs of the witch hazel tree, and is naturally astringent – making it great for oily or problem skins.

One ingredient you won't find in my recipes is lanolin. First, I'm sensitive to it; it makes my skin itch. Second, I would want to be absolutely sure that if I used lanolin, it came from organic sheep. Lanolin is derived from sheep's wool – and sheep are routinely dipped in toxic substances, including organophosphate pesticides. Those are not something I want anywhere near my skin, thanks.

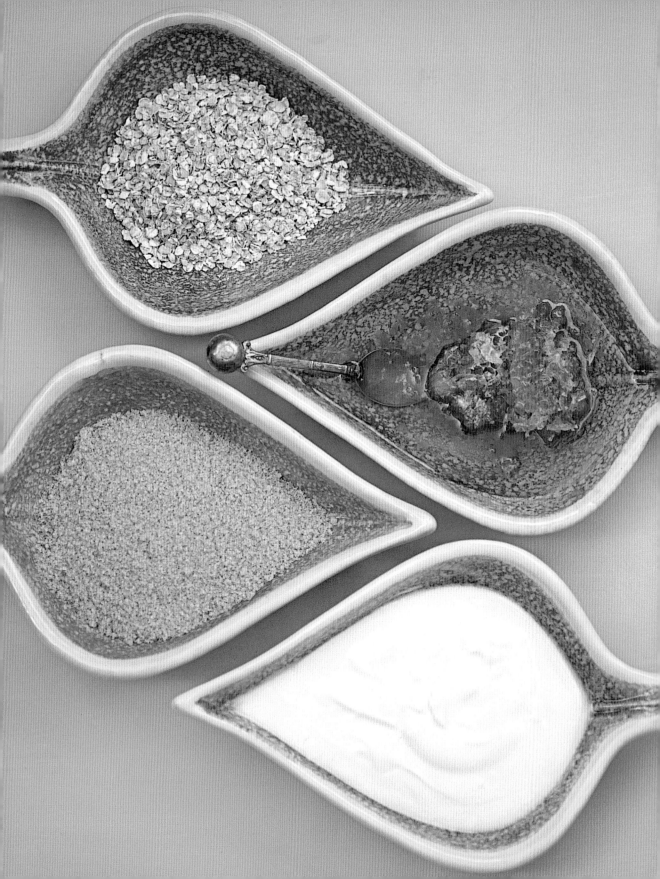

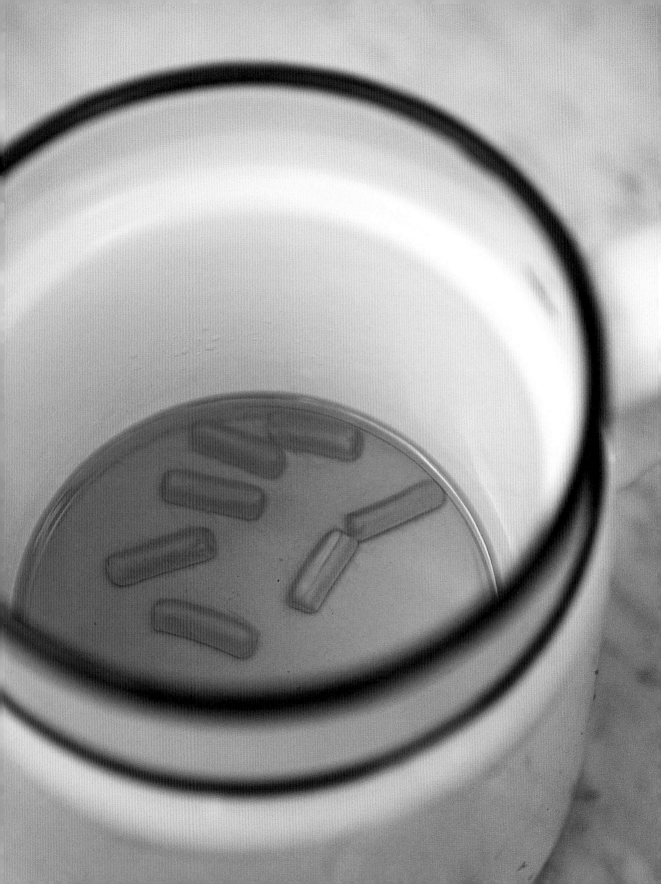

natural beauty techniques

Here are the very simple techniques I've referred to throughout the book which help you turn natural botanicals into skin-saving, hair-nourishing, body-smoothing treats.

How to use a double-boiler If you put oils or beeswax directly in a pan and heated them on the hob, they'd get too hot. So for making cosmetics – just as for melting chocolate – they need to be 'insulated' inside a double-boiler. The easiest thing to do is invest in a *bain marie* or double-boiler: one pan fits neatly inside the other, and a small quantity of water is placed in the outer pan; when this boils, it gently melts the ingredients inside the inner pan without spoiling them. If you don't have a double-boiler you can improvise with a pan and a smaller, Pyrex glass or a heatproof ceramic bowl which fits snugly inside: put about 2.5 cm/1 inch of boiling water in the bottom of the pan and place the heatproof bowl inside it. The heat from the water will melt and infuse any ingredients in the inner bowl. (NB If you use the bowl/pan technique, be extra careful not to be scalded by the steam, and take care not to burn yourself when removing the inner bowl.)

How to make a *tisane* (or **tea**) Use 1 teaspoon dried herb per 225ml (8fl oz) boiling water (or 1 teabag per cup if, say, you're making a chamomile *tisane*). Ideally, cover the cup – a saucer is ideal – or the volatile oils will be lost into the air while the tea steams. Steep for 10–15 minutes. Kept in the fridge, a *tisane* will keep for up to a week.

How to make an infusion Pour 600ml (1 pint) of boiling water over 25g (1oz) dried herbs and flowers and allow to steep for several hours (the difference between a *tisane* and an infusion is basically the length of time you leave the herbs to steep). Always make infusions in glass, stainless steel or enamel, never aluminium (as the herbs can leach out the metal). As with a *tisane*, an infusion will keep for up to 1 week in the fridge.

How to make a decoction Woodier herbs and hard seeds need to be boiled for longer to extract their potency. For each 25g (1oz) root, seed or bark, simmer in 600ml (1 pint) water for up to 1 hour over a low heat on the stove. (Again, always use stainless steel, glass or enamel pans.) Then let the pan sit for at least another hour, to allow the goodness of the herbs to disperse fully into the water.

NB As a rule of thumb, you should use approximately half the quantity of dried herbs as you would fresh in a decoction or *tisane*. You can also do this in a double-boiler if you're making a decoction using oils.

How to macerate oils All herbs should be chopped or ground. Dried herbs are better than fresh, for maceration. Submerge the herbs totally in oil, pushing them down, if necessary, otherwise mould may occur; tap the jar to see if you can get rid of any air bubbles that the plants may have trapped. (Do not wash the herbs, even if they may seem a little dusty.) Stand the jar in a warm, sunny place for at least 10 days and up to 3 weeks; you may want to stir or shake the contents gently daily. After the oils have macerated for long enough, strain them through a piece of muslin or a double layer of kitchen paper (which I find works just as well), pressing down with the back of a wooden spoon or gently with your fingers, to squeeze out the last of the goodness from the herbs. Macerated oils generally last from 6 months to a year.

resources

UK

Aveda

www.aveda.com

I've mentioned Aveda in the make-up chapter because if you are looking for natural make-up, theirs is 'greener' than most. They don't use petrochemical products – and are experimenting with natural pigments, including 'uruku' (used in lip, eye and cheek products), produced in collaboration with the indigenous Yawanawa tribe, in the Amazon.

G. Baldwin & Co.

171/173 Walworth Road, London SE17 1RW
+44 (0)20 7252 5550
www.baldwins.co.uk

Baldwins offer a good selection of jars and bottles (plastic and glass) as well as aromatherapy supplies, herbs, waxes and oils. They will ship all over the world.

Fragrant Earth

+44 (0)1485 831216
www.fragrant-earth.com

Fragrant Earth can supply many of the ingredients for this book – especially the oils and essential oils – and have distributors in many countries. Their website will indicate your nearest outlet/representative.

Dr Hauschka

+44 (0) 1386 792622
www.dr.hauschka.co.uk

Creators of some of the most natural make-up and skincare in the world, including a suberb range of mineral sunblocks.

Jane Iredale Mineral Make-up

+44 (0)20 8450 7111
www.janeiredale.com

This is one of the purest make-up ranges available anywhere in the world, created from mined mineral pigments. It is ideal for even the most sensitive skins (as it doesn't need preservatives), and is even recommended by cosmetic surgeons for patients to use to disguise scars soon after surgery. So it's very gentle indeed.

Jekka's Herb Farm

Rose Cottage, Shellards Lane, Alveston, Bristol BS35 3SY
www.jekkasherbfarm.com

I sourced all the herb plants that I used for this book from Jekka's Soil Association-certified nursery – and they were of superb quality. The herb seeds that Jekka offers can be shipped all over the world, and she offers a downloadable catalogue from her website. For anyone who wants to grow their own herbal and plant ingredients, I recommend her books on growing and using herbs, including *Jekka's Complete Herb Book*, which covers 355 different herbs from Aaron's root to Zingiber (ginger).

Liz Earle Naturally Active Skincare

+44 (0)1983 813913
www.lizearle.com

Liz uses high levels of botanical ingredients in her skincare, and offers a great mineral-based suncare range. The site will ship worldwide.

Neal's Yard Remedies

+44 (0)161 831 7875

www.nealsyardremedies.com

See website for shop locations

Neal's Yard Remedies are my No. 1 choice for home beauty supplies – because they offer the widest range of organically certified base oils, essential oils, dried herbs and other ingredients, like beeswax and clays. I can't recommend this range too highly. They have distributors in some countries around the world but will ship to anywhere from the UK site.

NHR Organic Oils

+44 (0)845-816 0195

www.nhrorganicoils.com

NHR also offers a selection of organic oils, which they will shop around the world.

Organic Herb Trading Co.

+44 (0)1823 401205

www.organicherbtrading.co.uk

The Organic Herb Trading Company imports and distributes dried organic herbs and spices to the UK (as well as some oils and shea/cocoa butter etc.), but is primarily a wholesaler – so you'll usually need to order in quantities of 1 kilo or more.

Spiezia Organics

+44 (0)1326 231600

www. spiezia.co.uk

The first range of fully organic skincare to be certified by The Soil Association; will ship worldwide.

USA AND CANADA

Aveda

www.aveda.com

See UK entry for comments

Camden Grey Essential Oils

(305) 500 9630

Toll free (877) 232 7662

www.camdengrey.com

A one-stop shop for essential oils (both organic and standard cultivation),base oils, salts, clays, bottles, lip balm containers, plus their exclusive LecheFresca™ bottle, which is like an old-fashioned US milk bottle (and ideal for making gifts of bath salts/lotions etc.).

Eco-natural.com

(250) 353 9680

www.eco-natural.com

This Canadian site offers organic and wild-crafted essential oils and base oils, as well as an unusually large range of Celtic sea salts that are perfect for making scrubs; will ship to the US and the rest of the world.

Dr Hauschka

(800) 247 9907

www.dr.hauschka.com

See UK entry for comments

Jane Iredale Mineral Make-up

www.janeiredale.com

In Canada, Jane Iredale is distributed by Stogryn Sales Ltd:
(800) 661 7024 www.stogryn.ca

Liz Earle Naturally Active Skincare

+44 (0) 1983 813913

www.lizearle.com

See UK entry for comments

Mountain Rose Herbs

(800) 879 3337

www.mountainroseherbs.com

This company prides itself on its ethical standards and offers a wide selection of organic products ideal for use in cosmetics, including clays, floral waters, butters, beeswax, base oils and essential oils, as well as jars/containers/sprays to put them in. They will ship internationally (call country code +541-741 7341).

Mulberry Creek

(419) 433 6126

www.mulberrycreek.com

This Ohio-based herb farm offers the largest selection of quality certified organic herbs in pots in the US, ideal for ground cover, culinary – and of course, cosmetic – uses.

Neal's Yard Remedies

Mail order catalogue: (888) 697 8721

www.nealsyardremediesusa.com

See UK entry for comments

In Canada, Neal's Yard Remedies are available through: Authentic Essence: (1) 416 769 6125 e-mail: riancassells@compuserve.com

NHR Organic Oils

(866) 816 0194

www.nhr.kz

See UK entry for comments

Sage Woman Herbs

www.sagewomanherbs.com

(719) 473 9702

A very wide selection of mail order herbs, base oils and other essential ingredients.

Spiezia Organics

+44 (0)1326 231600

www. spiezia.co.uk

See UK entry for comments

Sunrose Aromatics

(718) 794 0391

Toll Free (888) 382 9451

www.sunrosearomatics.com

An excellent selection of base oils, butters and aromatherapy ingredients (including a wide selection of organically certified essential oils). The site, which has won a couple of awards, also includes a selection of recipes for making your own cosmetics.

JAPAN

Aveda

www.aveda.com

See UK entry for comments

Jane Iredale

Jane Iredale is distributed by Medical Research International (MRI Inc.): (813) 5770 5415 www.mri-beauty.com

Neal's Yard Remedies

03-5778-3544

www.nealsyard.co.jp

AUSTRALIA

Allcrafts Goods & Services
(08) 9310 7884   e-mail: allcrafts@p085.aone.net.au
Supplies for hand-made soap and toiletries makers.

Aveda
www.aveda.com
See UK entry for comments

Jane Iredale
In Australia and New Zealand, contact Margifox Distributors:
(61) 01 3008 50008   e-mail: orders.mfd@bigpond.com

Green Harvest
1(800) 681 014
www.greenharvest.com.au
Suppliers of organic herb seeds and plants.

NEW ZEALAND
www.organicpathways.co.nz
A useful 'master site' which can help you track down
suppliers of organic herb plants, as well as oils, waxes etc.

Aveda
www.aveda.com
See UK entry for comments

Aromaflex
(03) 545 6217
www.aromaflex.co.nz
Offer a range of organic essential oils.

Jane Iredale
See Australia entry

GOOD WEBSITES

www.makeyourowncosmetics.com
If you sign up for their e-mailing list, you'll be sent a weekly
recipe to make at home.

**www.demoz.org/Shopping/Health/Alternative/
Bodycare_Products**
This is a good website which gives an overview of natural
ingredients and ready-made products that are available all
over the world.

**www.arhs.net/Shopping/Health/Alternative/
Aromatherapy/BodycareProducts**
Another 'overview' site with links to dozens of different
aromatherapy suppliers and natural beautycare companies.

www.mangobutter.com
This is a 'master site' with entries from hundreds of
different aromatherapy and cosmetic ingredients suppliers,
and is a great 'one-stop shop'.

www.myownlabels.com
This is a wonderful site if you want to personalise your
labels: they'll print any message you like on attractive, stick-
on labels (in a wide range of typefaces and designs), and
will ship anywhere in the world.

www.bellaonline.com
If you want to take what you've learned in this book a
stage further, this site offers an on-line course (price US
$20) with e-mail classes in making lip balms, hair care,
natural soaps, facial products etc.

www.world.std.com
Information about making your own perfumes, together
with a brief history of perfumery.

www.beautybible.com
Author's website.

index

botanical index

Further information about using plants can be found under their common names in the main index.